C0-ALR-901

Advances in Cardiovascular Nursing

Advances in Cardiovascular Nursing

Edward B. Diethrich, M.D.
President, Arizona Heart Institution Foundation

Robert J. Brady Co.
A Prentice-Hall Company

Advances in Cardiovascular Nursing

Copyright © 1979 by Robert J. Brady Co.
All rights reserved. No part of this publication may be reproduced or transmitted in any form or by any means, electronic or mechanical, including photocopying and recording, or by any information storage and retrieval system, without permission in writing from the publishers. For information, address Robert J. Brady Company, Bowie, Maryland 20715

Library of Congress Cataloging in Publication Data
Cardiovascular Nursing Symposium, 5th, Phoenix, Ariz.,
1978.
Advances in cardiovascular nursing.

Proceedings of the 5th annual Cardiovascular Nursing Symposium of the Arizona Heart Institute sponsored by the Arizona Heart Institute Foundation.
Bibliography: p.
Includes index.
1. Cardiovascular disease nursing--Congresses. I. Diethrich, Edward B. II. Arizona Heart Institute. III. Arizona Heart Institute Foundation. IV. Title. RC674.C37 1978   616.1   79-9375
ISBN 0-87619-457-9

Prentice-Hall International, Inc., London
Prentice-Hall of Australia, Pty., Ltd., Sydney
Prentice-Hall of India Private Limited, New Delhi
Prentice-Hall of Japan, Inc., Tokyo
Prentice-Hall of Southeast Asia Pte. Ltd., Singapore
Whitehall Books, Limited, Petone, New Zealand

Printed in the United States of America
79 80 81 82 83 84 85   10 9 8 7 6 5 4 3 2 1

RRATA SHEET

dvances in Cardiovascular Nursing

Contents

Contributors

Robert W. Barnes, MD
David Hume, Professor of Surgery
Medical Center of Virginia
Virginia Commonwealth University
Richmond, VA 23298

Larry Capps, BS
Exercise Physiologist
Arizona Heart Disease Foundation
Shalimar Medical Center
2034 E. Southern Avenue
Tempe, AZ 85282

Robert J. Clark, MD
Associate, Arizona Center for Chest Disease
2910 N. 3rd Street
Phoenix, AZ 85012

Sheila Coonen, RN, CVS
Nursing Supervisor, Cardiovascular Laboratory
Arizona Heart Institute
4800 N. 22nd Street
Phoenix, AZ 85016

Valerie Crain, RN
Supervisor, Ocular Pulse and Vascular Laboratory
Tucson Medical Center
PO Box 6067
Tucson, AZ 85733

G. A. Diamond, MD
Cedars-Sinai Medical Center
Los Angeles, CA 90029

Edward B. Diethrich, MD
Director, Arizona Heart Institute
4800 N. 22nd Street
Phoenix, AZ 85016

Jacklyn L. Ellis, RDMS
Ultrasound Technologist
Ultrasound Diagnostic Services
444 W. Osborn
Phoenix, AZ 85013

James S. Forrester, Jr., MD
Codirector, Specialized Center for Research
in Ischemic Heart Disease
Cedars-Sinai Medical Center
Los Angeles, CA 90029

Caroline M. Hughes, RN
Coordinator of Cardiopulmonary Rehabilitation
Scottsdale Memorial Hospital
7400 E. Osborn
Scottsdale, AZ 85251

Sam A. Kinard, MD
Chief of Cardiology
Arizona Heart Institute
4800 N. 22nd Street
Phoenix, AZ 85016

Edith M. McCarter, RN, CVS, MS
Director, Cardiovascular Nurse Specialist Program
Arizona Heart Institute
4800 N. 22nd Street
Phoenix, AZ 85016

Betty J. Phillips, RDMS
Ultrasound Technologist
Supervisor, Division of Cardiology
Ultrasound Diagnostic Services
444 W. Osborn
Phoenix, AZ 85013

Marilyn Reiling, RN, CVS, RT, BS
Supervisor, Peripheral Vascular Diagnostic Laboratory
Arizona Heart Institute
4800 N. 22nd Street
Phoenix, AZ 85016

Susan J. Sherbocker, RN, CVS
Nurse Therapist, Cardiopulmonary Rehabilitation
Scottsdale Memorial Hospital
7400 E. Osborn
Scottsdale, AZ 85251

John Stoner, MD
2 Palm Court
Menlo Park, CA 94025

RanVas, MD
Cedars-Sinai Medical Center
Los Angeles, CA 90029

Jack H. Wilmore, PhD
Chief, Department of Physical Education and Athletics
University of Arizona
Tucson, AZ 85721

Executive Producer — William Gibson
Book Design and Production — Laura Lammens

Foreword

No field of medicine demands more teamwork than the specialties of cardiovascular medicine and surgery. The days of a physician, surgeon, nurse or technician working independently on a patient suffering from cardiovascular disease are long past. The modern approach to cardiovascular diagnosis and care requires an integrated team in which each member understands not only his own function but also how those responsibilities relate to others. In the care of the patient, every member is equally important, for the chain of responsibility and trust between patient, physician and nurse must be sound if quality health care is to be provided. The key to assuring quality performance from each team member, and therefore from the team as a whole, is continual education in the newest techniques in cardiovascular care, with timely review of procedures less frequently used or less well understood.

In the realm of nursing education, the Arizona Heart Institute Foundation has met this challenge by sponsoring intensive, six-month, postgraduate training courses for nurses so they may become specialized in the care of the cardiac patient. These cardiovascular nurse specialists are thereafter qualified to establish their own teams and assume competent leadership roles. In addition the Foundation sponsors a yearly symposium at which these cardiovascular nurse specialists and other nurses working in the field meet and exchange ideas on topics of current interest and importance in cardiovascular nursing.

In this book are presented the papers which were given at the Fifth Annual Cardiovascular Nursing Symposium of the Arizona Heart Institute. As the topic of the conference, "Problems in Cardiovascular Nursing," reflects, this text is directed toward some of the more difficult areas of patient management in cardiovascular nursing. The new concepts, reviews and discussions contained on the following pages should offer an excellent opportunity for nurses in all areas of cardiovascular care to be made aware of the challenges present in the everyday care of the cardiac patient. These symposium papers provide an excellent update on the state of the art and clearly reflect the nursing profession's dedication toward the highest-quality patient care.

It has been a privilege for members of the Arizona Heart Institute's staff to participate in the preparation of this symposium. We trust that the entire nursing community will find the ideas presented at this meeting helpful.

Edward B. Diethrich, MD
President, Arizona Heart Institute Foundation

Introduction

Edith M. McCarter, RN, CVS, MS
Director, Cardiovascular
Nurse Specialist Program

According to 1977 statistics from the Amercan Heart Association, over 29,000,000 Americans have some form of heart and blood vessel disease. Included are those with hypertension, coronary heart disease, rheumatic heart disease and stroke. It is estimated that 52% of all deaths in 1977 were the result of cardiovascular disease. These figures attest to the magnitude of the problem and indicate why millions of dollars are spent annually on research related to prevention and treatment.

As nurses, we are involved in all phases of this fight against America's number one killer. One of our biggest challenges is keeping current. If we, indeed, want excellence in patient care as we profess, it is a challenge and commitment we each must actively strive to meet.

Let's look at the role of the cardiovascular nurse. Helen Creighton describes seven legal definitions of nursing which certainly apply to all of us.[1] We have a legal duty to observe, recognize and interpret symptoms and reactions. We must be able to recognize arrhythmias, Stokes-Adams attacks, dyspnea, and so forth, and act appropriately.

Another legal duty is that of accurately recording and reporting all significant information. Inherent in this responsibility are such things as knowing how to appropriately make corrections, noting the time the physician is notified of a particular patient problem, and making sure words are properly spelled. Carol Stadler, an attorney from Michigan who spoke at last year's symposium, stated that when a case is brought to court, regardless of the care given, she can tell whether the case will be won strictly on the basis of charting.

The third and fourth areas mentioned by Creighton can be combined. The nurse is responsible for carrying out requisite nursing functions with due care and also for carrying out physicians' orders and understanding why. Not infrequently, the problem confronts us of what's medicine and what's nursing? Many states are changing their Nurse Practice Acts to allow the nurse an expanded role. In critical care areas much of what we do, at least in an emergency situation, is covered by standing orders. Whatever the situation, know what you are allowed to do. And remember *you* are ultimately responsible for anything you do. Know when to question and when to refuse to implement an order. I'm sure many of us have been in a situation where a physician or someone else has said, "Go ahead — I'll take full responsibility." If you perform the act, you are responsible.

Another legal requirement is possessing the ability to use equipment properly and to recognize when it's malfunctioning. This is particularly applicable in a critical care area with all of the advanced technology.

Supervision of others under your professional level who are involved in patient care is still another legal responsibility. This means LPNs, nursing students, nursing assistants, etc. Making sure assignments are within the scope of the person's education and experience is essential in assuring quality patient care.

The seventh responsibility involves patient teaching. This has long been a controversial subject. Some physicians do not want nurses teaching their patients for several probable reasons — the historically subservient role of nurses, inaccurate information given to patients by nurses, desire of the physician to remain totally in control of all aspects of patient care. Whatever the reason, nurses are becoming more involved and, in fact, are legally responsible for some patient teaching. Teaching is so important for the cardiovascular patient who needs to know about risk factors, medications and activity. But there's more than just *patient* teaching. Why wait for an individual to assume a patient role? Preventive medicine is a whole new field that nurses certainly are becoming involved in. Why not put more emphasis on health education beginning in the young school age population? We're seeing screening clinics for hypertension and diabetes. Prevention and early detection depend on public awareness — nurses can play a key role.

Contingent upon performing the above duties is keeping current, a commitment we must all make. What a challenge! The nurse's role has changed dramatically in recent years and will continue to do so as we enlarge our knowledge base and sharpen clinical skills. Nurses weren't allowed to take a patient's blood pressure as recently as 1940. Today we're not only measuring traditional vital signs but also assessing patients via sophisticated monitoring tools. Gone are the days of being a passive member of the health-care team. We seek to be active participants in the delivery of health care, to make independent decisions. We must make sure we're ready. The responsibility of continually learning and applying new information, in addition to remembering the old, can sometimes be overwhelming and frustrating. But it's also one of the exciting challenges of being a nurse.

What are some of the new things we've been exposed to in the last few years? Many things come to mind — the Swan Ganz catheter and intra-aortic balloon pump; drugs such as intropin, norpace, and nipride; the Doppler exam, oculoplethysmography (OPG), and carotid phonoangiography (CPA) for screening peripheral disease; new concepts about myocardial preservation; use of the porcine valve; more aggressive ideas about conditioning for cardiovascular patients. The latest on many of these subjects and more will be presented to you in group sessions and also through materials at our learning resource center. What will the next year, five, ten years bring in the field of cardiovascular nursing? Many exciting things, we can be sure.

How do we keep current? Some believe mandatory continuing education is the answer. This is certainly an issue currently facing us in nursing. Do you, as a professional, know the pros and cons of this issue? The consumer is demanding that he has a right to safe and up-to-date care; hopefully, as care givers, we believe that also. But should we have to be told that our education must continue in order to help keep us updated? As professionals, should we not be responsible for our own professional growth and destiny? Many nurses do, of course, feel this responsibility. Certainly there are many other ways of gaining new information — attending hospital inservices and conferences, reading professional literature, working at the bedside. The key is motivation, interest, a commitment to learn. And, of course, once the information is acquired, it must be clinically applied. Putting theory into practice is sometimes the most difficult part. But, oh, how important! We all know that it takes more than intelligence to be a good nurse.

I think we all have our own picture of the "ideal nurse" — our role model. It's been said that there are four types of nurses — the "wishbones," who spend their time wishing someone would do the work; the "jawbones," who do all the talking but very little else; the "knucklebones," who knock everything that anyone tries to do; and the "backbones," who get under the load and do the work. Hopefully, our role model would fit into this latter category. On a more serious note, what are some other qualities that we look for — expert clinical competence, good decision-making ability, resourcefulness and ingenuity, effective communication skills, ability to readily adapt to the unexpected and unusual. The list could go on and on. The important point is that each of us is a role model to someone else. We are influenced by how others act and look; we, in turn, influence others. This certainly has implication on a professional level. Commitment to excellence, intellectual curiosity, and expert practice help to stimulate these same traits in our co-workers. Robert F. Kennedy once said, "Few will have the greatness to bend history itself, but each of us can work to change a small portion of events and in the total of all those acts will be written the history of this generation." Let us not forget the impact we can have.

We've talked about duties, responsibilities, the pressure to keep up-to-date — what an awesome task. Sometimes, we feel like "What's the use? Why bother?" I think the answer for most of us is that we care; we care about people, our patients, our students, our colleagues. What personal reward and satisfaction to know we've done something to help another! The frustrations, anxieties, the physical tiredness of the effort are overwhelmed by the sense of accomplishment when we see positive results — the critical patient who progresses from the intensive care unit (ICU) to a general floor; the pacemaker patient who, after repeated instruction, can accurately count his pulse; the family member who, after losing a loved one, says, "thank you" for all you've done. These are gratifying incidents, but we all know it's not always like that.

It costs to care. As I once heard it put, "What do we do when we get sick and tired of caring for the tired and sick?" Psychologists write about emotional burnout. Members of high-stress, high-human-contact occupations — policemen, prison guards, welfare workers, doctors, nurses — are especially subject to emotional burnout. Dr. Christina Maslach, from San Francisco, describes it in this way:

> When you burn out, your emotional center goes. There's nothing that you really care about. You don't have any optimistic feelings, only negative ones. You don't like people you work with and wish they'd go away. You treat them in institutional, routinized, dehumanizing ways.[2]

Dr. Maslach goes on to say that those who can cope best are those who can separate their personal and professional lives. They can leave work at work. One can't avoid stress, whether professional or personal, in today's world. I don't think we would really want to. A certain amount of stress stimulates us to perform at an optimum level. It's when the stresses become excessive and unconquerable that one is subject to emotional burnout. This can be avoided by periodically taking time to recharge our emotions, to reflect, to reevaluate, to set new goals.

In conclusion, we all know there are costs and responsibilities in any profession. Cardiovascular nursing isn't unique in that respect. What is unique are the rewards and challenges. Indeed, it's an exciting time as we open this, our fifth symposium, and look at some of the challenges facing us. Welcome to Problems: Current Challenges in Cardiovascular Nursing.

REFERENCES

1.   Creighton Helen. Your legal risks in nursing coronary patients — how you can (and should) minimize them. Nursing '77, pp 65-68, January, 1977.

2.   Putney Michael. Burnout: A high price for caring. The National Observer, p 14, July 11, 1977.

Section 1

Ultrasonography and Real-Time Imaging

Often in our history, we have taken a theory or technique developed for one application and adapted it to an entirely new situation. So the use of ultrasound, sound waves above the audible range, began as sonar in World War II. In the 1950s, however, scientists recognized the potential which ultrasonics had in medicine. Since that time, the use of ultrasound has broadened from therapeutic applications to its more widely known diagnostic uses.

In cardiovascular medicine, ultrasonography, otherwise known as echocardiography when used on the heart, has been employed for a decade or more as a means of viewing the cardiac structures, particularly the valves. Of late, rapid technological developments in instrumentation have greatly enhanced the diagnostic capabilities of echocardiography. With the advent of two-dimensional scanning, the motion of the heart in a two-dimensional, real-time mode can now be visualized.

Improvements in equipment and technique have also made possible real-time ultrasonic scanning of the entire abdominal aorta and its branches, when just a few years ago, ultrasound examination of the abdomen could detect only aortic aneurysms. Now this much more complete picture of the vessel walls and branches can help locate and define atheromas in the aortic tree.

The paper on ultrasound is a comprehensive review and discussion of ultrasonographic principles, equipment, and diagnostic testing. It offers an excellent outline of ultrasound's applicability to cardiovascular diagnosis and introduces the latest innovations in technology.

The Role of Ultrasound in Cardiovascular Diagnostic Medicine

Jacklyn L. Ellis, RDMS, and Betty J. Phillips, RDMS

In the area of cardiovascular diagnostic medicine, ultrasound is a well documented and accepted procedure. In an increasing number of clinical situations it is considered essential for patient care. The procedure is harmless and noninvasive and there is no evidence that ultrasound at the frequencies used for diagnostic procedures damages biological tissue or constitutes any hazard to human health.

Ultrasound was developed as early as World War I and was actively employed during World War II in the form of SONAR to locate enemy submarines. A crystal was submerged in water and stimulated by an electrical charge. The same crystal not only had the capability of sending the sound, but could also receive it. A beam was sent out and then, in effect, listened for. The equipment kept track of the total time the beam of sound took to travel to the object, to reflect off the object and return back to the crystal. Because the speed of sound in fluid is constant, the depth of the reflecting object could be calculated (Figure 1.1).

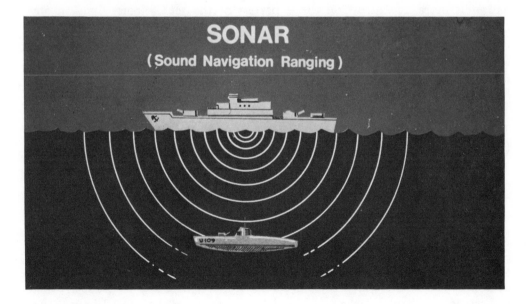

FIGURE 1.1   Sound waves transmitted from a crystal submerged in water can track the speed and the depth of the objects along its beam path.

It was with these same principles in mind that medical researchers first applied ultrasound to the field of diagnostic medicine. They found that sound waves with a frequency of one million cycles per second (one megahertz) or more allowed for visualization of internal organs and soft tissue. Just as the sound waves bounced off the objects hidden beneath the ocean, they, too, bounce off the internal structures of the body.

Since that time, many advancements have been made in the electronics that control the ultrasound image, although the basic principles remain very much the same.

M-MODE ECHOCARDIOGRAM

The standard m-mode (time-motion mode) echocardiogram is presently the most widely used ultrasound method in the examination of the internal structures of the heart. It depicts the movement of the cardiac valves, the septum, the ventricles and the atria throughout the cardiac cycle. The echocardiogram can provide evidence of valvular heart disease, congenital heart disease, hypertensive cardiovascular disease and coronary artery disease.

The examination should be performed by a qualified technologist or physician. The clinician must be knowledgeable about cardiac anatomy and the normal and abnormal physiology of the cardiac structures. The importance of this cannot be overly stressed. The quality of the echocardiographic examination is more dependent on the expertise of the technologist than on any other single factor. A technologist who is not thoroughly acquainted with echocardiography will tend to underestimate both its difficulties and the enormous extent of its applications. Technical errors can easily be produced, making accurate interpretation by the physician extremely difficult, if not impossible.

No patient preparation is needed for the echocardiographic procedure. The patient is examined in the supine or rolled onto the left lateral position (Figure 1.2). There is no discomfort to the patient during the examination, which routinely takes approximately one-half hour to perform.

In performing the examination, a small probe or *transducer* is placed on the anterior surface of the chest at approximately the third, fourth or fifth intercostal space, just to the left of the sternum. This area is referred to as the *cardiac window*, as it is generally the location where penetration of the sound beam will not be obstructed by overlying lung tissue or bone. Lung tissue absorbs and scatters the sound waves. Bone prevents penetration of the sound beam and creates a similar barrier, thus the transducer signal is directed between the ribs and lung in order to enter the heart (Figure 1.3). Clear recordings are difficult to perform on patients with chronic obstruc-

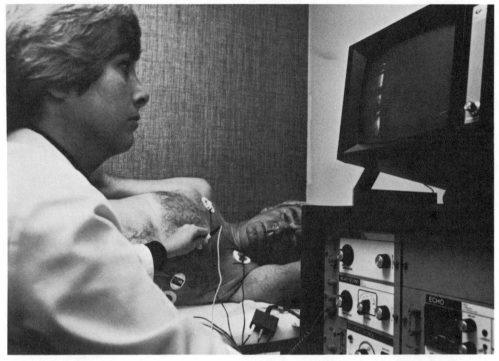

FIGURE 1.2   The standard echocardiogram is performed usually with the patient in the left lateral position. The transducer is placed at approximately the level of the fourth intercostal space and directed through the ribs and into the heart.

tive lung disease as the cardiac window is usually covered by overlying lung tissue.

The width of the sound beam varies slightly but usually is about one inch in diameter. Thus a limitation of the m-mode is that only a narrow segment of the heart is visualized at any given moment and the interrelationships of the cardiac structures are sometimes difficult to evaluate (Figure 1.4).

When the area of interest is identified by the signal complexes seen on the oscilloscope, the operator records the information on a strip-chart recorder. The strip-chart recorder enables the operator to record long strips of uninterrupted data such as the opening and closing motion of the valves as well as heart-wall contraction, wall thickness and chamber size. Depth is plotted vertically and time is plotted horizontally. A simultaneous electrocardiogram is recorded to aid in the proper interpretation of the echocardiographic structures in the presence of any rhythm disturbances.

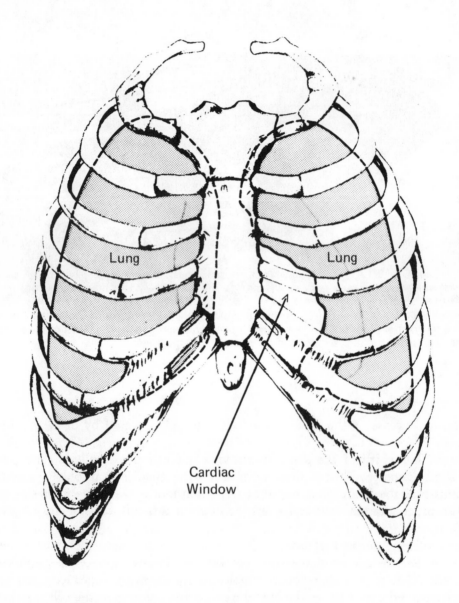

FIGURE 1.3   The sound beam is directed between the ribs in the area of the cardiac window (arrow) to avoid overlying lung tissue.

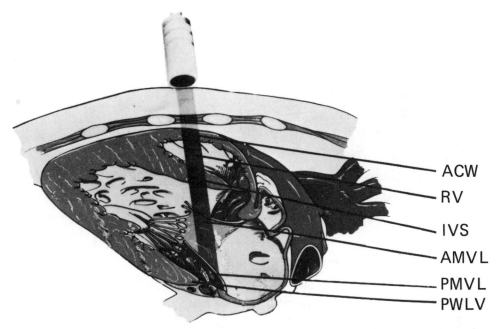

ACW
RV
IVS
AMVL
PMVL
PWLV

FIGURE 1.4   The single element transducer emits a relatively narrow sound beam which enables only a small segment of the heart in line with the beam path to be visualized at any given moment. (ACW = anterior chest wall; RV = right ventricle; IVS = interventricular septum; AMVL = anterior mitral valve leaflet; PMVL = posterior mitral valve leaflet; PWLV = posterior wall of left ventricle).

THE MITRAL VALVE

The mitral valve is one of the easiest of the cardiac structures to identify and has supplied investigators with the largest amount of diagnostic information. In recording the mitral valve, the ultrasound beam passes sequentially through the anterior heart wall, the right ventricular cavity, the interventricular septum, the left ventricular outflow tract, the anterior mitral valve leaflet, the posterior mitral valve leaflet, and exits through the posterior wall of the left ventricle (Figure 1.5).

Each phase of the motion of the mitral valve has been identified by letters A–F of the alphabet for purposes of diagnostic measurements and reference (Figure 1.6). Beginning in systole, the entire heart moves anteriorly during which time the mitral valve is in its closed position. With the onset of diastole (D point) during the period of rapid ventricular filling, the anterior and posterior leaflets of the mitral valve separate to their maximal opening (E point). After this initial filling period of the left ventricle, the anterior leaf-

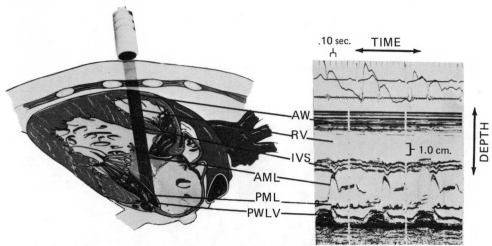

FIGURE 1.5   When directed through the heart toward the mitral valve leaflets, the sound beam passes sequentially through the anterior heart wall (AW), the right ventricle (RV), the interventricular septum (IVS), and through the left ventricular outflow tract. It then strikes the anterior mitral leaflet (AML), the posterior mitral leaflet (PML), and the posterior wall of the left ventricle (PWLV). Note that the depth markers are one centimeter apart (arrow).

let exhibits a rapid posterior movement to the F point which represents semiclosure. The E−F distolic descent slope represents the rate of left ventricular filling during diastole and is an important indicator of mitral valve disease. Following the P wave of the electrocardiogram, the left atrium contracts and the valve reopens to the A point, which normally exhibits only about two-thirds of the excursion exhibited by the E point. Immediately following the A point, valve closure begins and closes totally at the C point, corresponding with the QRS complex of the electrocardiogram.

In the presence of mitral stenosis where the leaflets are thickened and less pliable, the E−F slope is markedly reduced and the A wave is generally absent (Figure 1.7). In many cases of mitral stenosis, the echocardiogram is especially helpful in evaluating the pliability of the valve and in determining whether the patient is a candidate for commissurotomy or mitral valve replacement.

M-MODE APPLICATIONS

By slightly changing the angulation of the transducer from the mitral valve position, other cardiac structures can be visualized and recorded (Figure 1.8). Directing the transducer superiorly from the mitral valve, the ultrasound beam passes through the right side of the heart, the aortic root and the

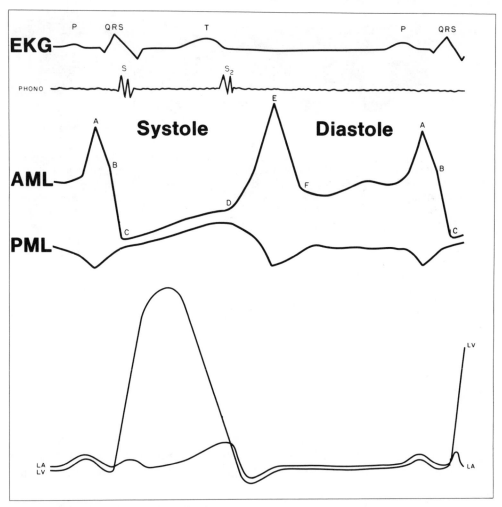

FIGURE 1.6   The phases of mitral valve motion as shown in relation to the cardiac cycle, phonocardiogram, and the left atrial and left ventricular pressure curves.

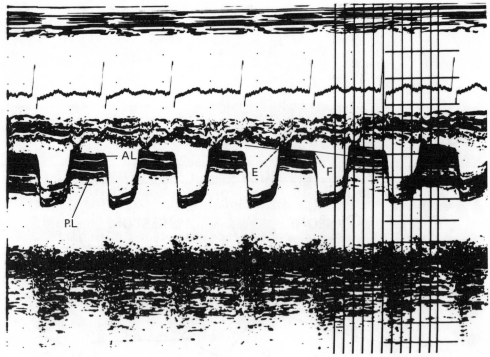

FIGURE 1.7   M-mode recording of a patient with mitral stenosis. The E-F slope (line) and/or rate of ventricular filling is considerably reduced measuring approximately 3mm/sec. Note that the posterior leaflet of the mitral valve (PL) moves anteriorly with the anterior mitral leaflet (AL). Both leaflets appear thickened and move in an abnormal fashion.

left atrium. Directing the transducer inferiorly and laterally from the mitral valve allows visualization of the left ventricle seen just below the mitral valve leaflets.

The list of clinical applications for the standard m-mode echocardiogram is long and continues to grow. It is for this reason that we have in this paper limited the discussion of these applications to only a few representative examples.

The echocardiogram may be helpful in assessing the significance of a heart murmur. An increasingly large number of patients are being evaluated for the *click-murmur* syndrome or prolapsing mitral valve. In the presence of mitral valve prolapse, one or both leaflets will bulge slightly into the area of the left atrium during systole. This is represented on the m-mode tracing as a posterior bowing of the leaflets after the point of mitral closure during ventricular systole (Figure 1.9).

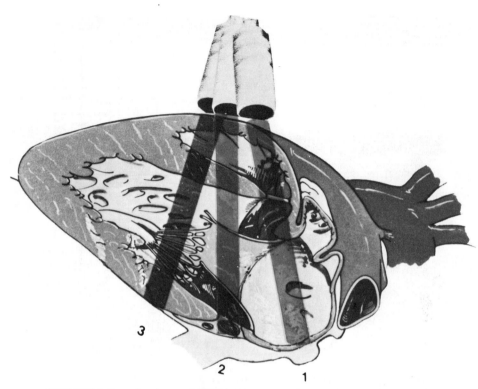

FIGURE 1.8   As the angle of the transducer is changed, the sound beam passes through different cardiac structures. In position (1), the sound beam passes through the aortic valve and the left atrium. In position (2), the motion of the mitral valve is visualized and in position (3), the sound beam passes through the right ventricle, interventricular septum, left ventricle, and posterior left ventricular wall.

Another primary application of the echocardiogram is in the detection of pericardial fluid. The presence of pericardial fluid can be easily identified on the m-mode tracing as an echo-free space located between the endocardium and the pericardium of the posterior wall of the left ventricle (Figure 1.10). With the patient who presents with an enlarged heart on x ray, echocardiography is of great value in differentiating between cardiomegaly and the presence of pericardial fluid.

TWO-DIMENSIONAL ULTRASOUND

One of the most recent advancements in cardiac ultrasound is the use of two-dimensional or real-time systems for viewing the cardiovascular structures. When used in conjunction with standard m-mode echocardiography,

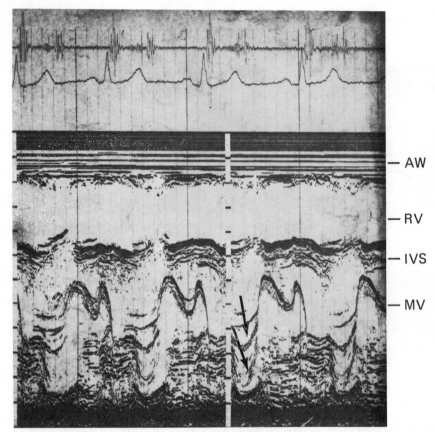

— AW

— RV

— IVS

— MV

FIGURE 1.9   M-mode recording representing mitral valve prolapse. During late systole, both the anterior and posterior mitral valve leaflets display a posterior bowing motion (arrows). (AW = anterior heart wall; RV = right ventricle; IVS = interventricular septum; MV=mitral valve).

real-time ultrasound offers the capability of greatly extending the means by which the heart can be studied noninvasively. Studies using angiography indicate that the left ventricle, for example, undergoes complex movements in three dimensions during its contraction. Data from a one-dimensional recording such as the m-mode does not faithfully capture all of these movements. Mainly because of its wide field of view and its ability to visualize moving structures, the two-dimensional system optimally allows for continuous observation of the dynamic motion of the entire cardiac anatomy. Individual structures are easily identified in both the longitudinal and transverse axis and the interrelationship of each structure can be assessed.

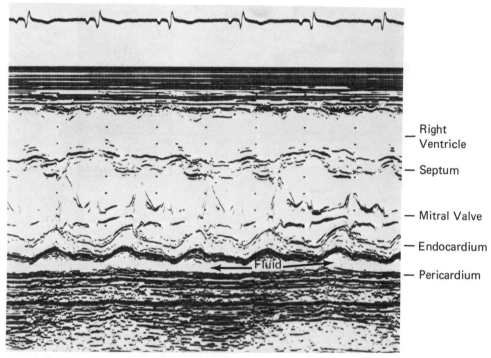

Right
Ventricle

— Septum

— Mitral Valve

— Endocardium

— Pericardium

Fluid

FIGURE 1.10 M-mode recording of a patient with a moderate degree of pericardial fluid. This fluid is represented by a clear echo-free space (arrow) seen between the
endocardium and pericardium.

Currently there are three major real-time systems available: the linear
array, the phased array, and the sector scanner. In the linear array system,
many small transducer elements (approximately 64) are mounted in a row and
fired sequentially at a very fast frame rate. The beam of sound is perpendicu-
lar to the elements and is moved along the array by electronic shifting of the
crystals. The result is a motion picture effect of a cross section approximately
2 cm wide by 10 cm long of the structures beneath the transducer (Figure
1.11).

Presently several limitations exist with this system that prohibit routine
observation of adult hearts. As previously discussed, bone blocks the transmission of sound. Thus when the transducer array is placed on the chest over
the area of the heart, the ribs obstruct a good portion of the area of interest.
This system, therefore, is not the instrument of choice for the adult heart, but
is more applicable in infants and small children or in viewing vascular structures such as the abdominal aorta or the carotid arteries.

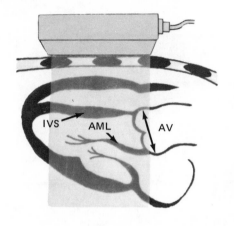
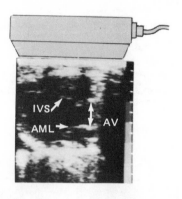

A   **B**

FIGURE 1.11   (A) Schematic representation of a linear array showing the beam pattern through the heart. (IVS = interventricular septum; AML = anterior mitral leaflet; AV = aortic valve). (B) Freeze-frame representation of a "real-time" linear array image of the segment shown in (A). Due to rib shadowing portions of the image are not clearly visualized (IVS = interventricular septum; AML = anterior mitral leaflet; AV = aortic valve).

By placing the linear array transducer along the midline of the abdomen, the pulsations from the abdominal aorta can be immediately viewed on the oscilloscope and traced along its course through the abdomen .(Figure 1.12). Any areas of dilation, calcification or dissection can be observed and recorded (Figure 1.13). The size and extent of any aneurysmal dilations can be measured and the presence of clot formation identified. Serial scans can be performed to follow any disease progression as the test is noninvasive and a relatively easy procedure for the patient.

Another application currently being evaluated is in the use of higher frequency linear array transducers for evaluation of the carotid arteries. The higher frequency transducer enables the carotid arteries to be localized and traced to the point of bifurcation (Figure 1.14). Preliminary studies on a relatively small number of patients have shown this application to have some promise. However, problems with instrumentation design combined with the physical properties affecting sound transmission in dealing with structures located close to the skin surface have produced some false results. Further development of this application will be necessary before this technique can be utilized as a routine diagnostic procedure.

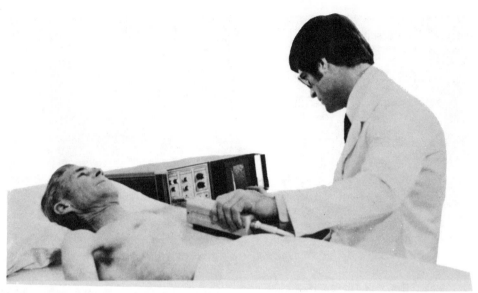

FIGURE 1.12 Transducer is placed (linear array real-time) over the long axis of the abdominal aorta. The ultrasound image of the vessel is viewed by the operator on the oscilloscope.

PHASED ARRAY SYSTEM

The phased array scanner consists of a hand-held array measuring approximately 2.4 cm in length and contains approximately 16 transducer elements. This system was specifically designed for cardiac applications and has overcome most of the limitations of the linear array design. By electronically phasing or timing the delay in the individual transducer crystals, the beam angle is altered or steered through the ribs and produces an imaged plane of a sector arc of up to 90°. The data is presented as a pie-shaped image which is narrow as it enters the right side of the heart and spreads to a wider view as it passes through the left side. The scanning process of this system is computerized and lends itself to future expansion by the use of different programs written for a wide variety of clinical situations. Currently its cost is considerably more than that of the other types of two-dimensional systems, making its use somewhat limited.

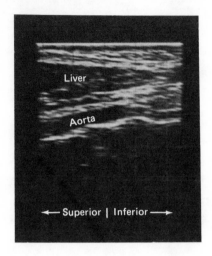
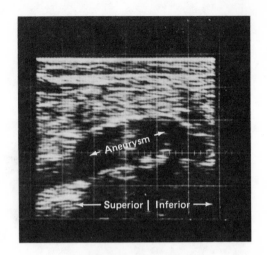

| A | B |

FIGURE 1.13 (A) Real-time linear array still photo of a normal abdominal aorta shown beneath the liver. (B) Real-time linear array still photo of an abdominal aortic aneurysm.

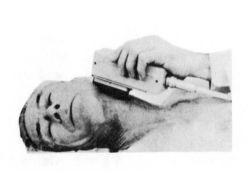
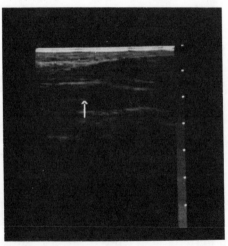

| A | B |

FIGURE 1.14 (A) A 7.0 MHz linear array transducer is placed on the neck along the longitudinal axis of the left carotid artery. (B) Ultrasound image of the left carotid artery showing the point of bifurcation (arrow).

MECHANICAL SECTOR SCANNER

The mechanical scanner, like the phased array, produces a pie-shaped image. The transducer, however, is composed of a single crystal which emits a real-time image by mechanically oscillating the transducer head very rapidly between the intercostal space (Figure 1.15). To date most of the current work has been produced with an image plane of a 30° arc but probes with arcs of up to 80° are now being made available. The wider arc will allow for broader sections of the heart to be viewed at one time. Data from these real-time sector scanners are videotaped for playback analysis and for permanent records. Slow motion and freeze frame capabilities of the video equipment allow for close observation of the cardiac structures and for quantitative measurements such as that of the mitral valve orifice and the long and transverse axis of the left ventricle.

In the field of noninvasive medicine, two-dimensional ultrasound presents itself as one of the most powerful and promising of the techniques being used to meet the challenges in cardiovascular disease today.

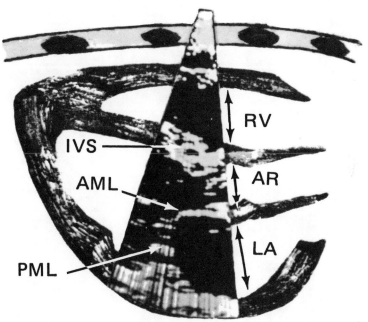

FIGURE 1.15   A two-dimensional 30° sector image of the heart showing the right ventricle (RV), the interventricular septum (IVS), aortic root (AR), aortic valve (AV), anterior mitral leaflet (AML), and posterior mitral leaflet (PML).

Section 2

Stress Electrocardiography

Exercise electrocardiography has risen to a place of considerable importance among the diagnostic tests which the cardiologist has at his disposal to evaluate patients with known or suspected coronary artery disease. Moreover the procedure is gaining wide acceptance as a screening procedure for the asymptomatic population to identify those people suffering from "silent" ischemia or functional difficulties.

Despite the popularity of this testing mode, there are still problems which must be resolved. The diagnostic criteria for the exercise test are not uniformly accepted by all diagnosticians. Debate still wages over the type, duration, and depth of ST segment alterations which would indicate a positive test. The test's validity and reliability are also impacted by this disagreement on interpretive criteria. Reports are being made on new studies which may help to shed light on the true prognostic significance of the test.

The papers in this section provide a rather complete review of the state of the art in exercise electrocardiography, covering the indications, contraindications, testing protocols, and complications which the nurse specialist should know. Two of the papers discuss interpretation of the stress electrocardiogram: one outlines the interpretation process and currently used criteria while the second investigates the question of false test results. Moreover, there is a discussion of the impact recent statistical correlations have had on the prognostic capacities of the stress test.

Indications and Contraindications for Stress Testing

Sheila Coonen, RN, CVS

Today, the most widely accepted means of exercise stress testing is the multi-stage treadmill test. Since its introduction in 1956 by Dr. Bruce, it has become the most frequently used noninvasive test for detecting coronary heart disease and assessing its severity. The reason it gained popularity so quickly was its reliability in predicting this disease.

In the symptomatic population, the predictive value of the stress test is high. According to a recent study, a patient with a normal resting electrocardiogram (ECG), no resting repolarization changes, exercise-induced chest pain and abnormal repolarization changes with exercise can be expected to have significant coronary artery disease with a 95% predictive accuracy.[1]

As stress testing criteria become more accurately defined, this test will become more valuable as a screening tool for asymptomatic people as well. However, Faris and associates at the Krannert Institute of Cardiology feel exercise screening of the asymptomatic population should be reserved for those subjects thought to be at greatest risk, based on other clinical criteria.[1] This may be a valid statement as it relates to uncovering an impaired coronary circulation; however, it does exclude the use of a stress test for evaluation of exercise tolerance, an application for which it is most valuable.

Since the preponderance of data regarding stress testing has been accumulated from the symptomatic, hospitalized population,[1] it is not feasible to apply the resultant statistics to the general populace. Therefore, the cardiologist evaluating a patient's symptoms must be constantly mindful of that patient's symptoms and history in order to adequately assess the response to exercise.

The six most common reasons for stress testing a person are: to discover latent coronary artery disease, to diagnose suspected coronary artery disease, to evaluate the degree of dysfunction, to evaluate therapy, to predict exercise capacity, and to motivate patients toward improving their life style. Those people at risk of developing coronary artery disease by virtue of their life style, heredity, or physical condition are primary candidates for exercise testing. Early detection of coronary artery disease is vitally important to the patient's survival, and although the stress test is not 100% accurate, it is nonetheless the best noninvasive tool for screening these high-risk people. Just as important is its applicability to anginal patients and those with atypical chest pain. Preliminary assessment of the cause of the pain is best conducted using the stress test.

Much information on a patient's condition can be obtained by an alert technician administering the test. Signs of cerebral anoxia (ataxic gait, confusion, visual disturbances), peripheral vascular occlusive disease (hip or calf pain, limping), or anxiety will aid the physician in his diagnosis. An episode of chest pain experienced on the treatmill can often be assigned to coronary ischemia by observing the typical anginal signs.[2]

Using the stress test to evaluate the degree of dysfunction a patient experiences applies to both cardiac and noncardiac conditions. It is common to employ a stress test in patients with valvular disease, pulmonary disease, arrhythmias, and so forth, to ascertain their maximum work level. On occasion, a person may be employed in a job which demands more of him physically than he can give, such as coordination or endurance. By using the results of a stress test, the cardiologist can prescribe an appropriate work level or determine when a person can return to his job.

It is not uncommon to evaluate medical or surgical therapy by stress testing a patient. The effectiveness of an antihypertensive regimen in a labile hypertensive patient can be assessed, as can the increase in exercise tolerance by an anginal patient recently placed on antiarrhythmic medication. Moreover, pre- and postoperative stress tests provide a great deal of information to the surgeon when evaluating the efficacy of an operative procedure. At the Arizona Heart Institute, most coronary artery bypass patients are stress tested two weeks following surgery. Although they are sore and perhaps anemic, improvement is noted in tolerance, ST segment depression, arrhythmias, and intensity or presence of pain. Since the atherosclerotic disease process may continue to affect coronary vessels even after operation, yearly reevaluation is conducted to monitor disease progression and graft patency.

In the postmyocardial infarction (MI) or postsurgical patient, an accurate assessment of work capacity is necessary before returning to a strenuous job or beginning a conditioning program. For this purpose, the exercise test is vital. By stress testing a patient to a symptom-limited maximum work tolerance level, various conditioning parameters can be calculated, such as target met (work) levels and heart rates. From these parameters, a work prescription can be written so that the person knows with confidence what he can and cannot do. For the post-MI or postsurgical patient, a safe work load is usually considered to be 70% of his maximum work capacity.

Lastly, among the indications for stress testing is its use as a motivating tool. One of the more serious problems in patients with coronary artery disease is motivating them toward improving their life style by removing such risk factors as obesity, smoking, stress, hypertension, inactivity, and hypercholesterolemia.[2] For many people, this entails a complete change in life style. One particularly helpful method of motivating these people is to compare their stress test results with those of a healthy individual of the same or greater

22

age in the hope that the detrimental effects of their current life style will be made apparent to them. By the same token, serial treadmill tests on patients in a conditioning program or ones who are altering their habits have a positive reinforcing effect.

As concerns the contraindications for stress testing, some cardiologists prefer to give absolute and relative contraindications. Of the former type, acute myocardial infarction, congestive heart failure, and unstable angina are agreed upon by most cardiologists. The relative contraindications are rapid atrial or ventricular arrhythmias, second- or third-degree heart block, high-grade left main coronary artery lesion or its equivalent, severe valvular disease, acute illness, and cardiovascular drug toxicity. These latter conditions may contraindicate a stress test at the physician's discretion, depending upon severity of symptoms and their resultant limitations.

In conclusion, the stress test is a valuable noninvasive tool for detecting and diagnosing coronary artery disease, assessing exercise tolerance levels, and evaluating dysfunction and therapeutic measures. With proper pretesting physician evaluation and well trained testing supervisors, the exercise test can be a highly accurate, safe diagnostic method.

REFERENCES

1. Faris, JV, McHenry, DL, Morris, SN: Concepts and applications of treadmill exercise testing and the exercise electrocardiogram. Amer Heart J 95:102-14, 1978.

2. Ellestad, MH: Stress Testing. Principles and Practice, Philadelphia, PA Davis, 1975.

Clinical Complications in Stress Testing

Larry Capps, BS

As anyone who has worked in a stress lab is aware, a multitude of items can occur to impair or destroy the validity of an exercise tolerance test. Equipment difficulties and physical limitations are by far the most frequently incurred complications.

It would be impossible and of little worth to individually treat each situation that might arise. Instead, an understanding of the basic principles of exercise physiology[4] and their proper application to the field of stress testing would enable each problem to be dealt with quickly and in a manner which leaves the validity of the test intact.

INDICATIONS FOR STRESS TESTING

A stress test may be required for any of four reasons:[1,8,16]

1) As an aid in the diagnosis of cardiovascular disorders.

2) To determine functional aerobic impairment which may be associated with coronary artery disease (CAD), myocardial infarction (MI), or deconditioning.

3) To identify safe levels of exercise for individuals suffering from CAD, MI or deconditioning.

4) To evaluate the efficaciousness of medications or a conditioning program.

For the purposes of this discussion, these four reasons will be reduced to two: tests for function and tests for diagnosis.[2]

OXYGEN CONSUMPTION AND EXERCISE

A stress test should be constructed so as to elicit a gradual increase in oxygen consumption[1,2,8,16,19] until the desired endpoint is obtained. This response is necessary for the test to have value. Knowledge of the aerobic principles of exercise testing is essential to design a protocol that will both satisfy the purpose of the test and accommodate the physical limitations of the patient. The American Heart Association in *A Handbook for Physicians* stated, "Exercise tests are standardized in terms of the oxygen cost associated with a specific task. Standardization is established by determining or estimating the oxygen uptake per unit of body weight; i.e., ml O_2/kg/min for each work level." If the O_2 uptake at a given level of work is divided by the O_2 required at rest, a unit called the MET is obtained. The MET is commonly used to describe work intensities or capacities encountered in exercise and in stress testing. The O_2 requirement at rest is generally assumed to be 3.5 ml O_2/kg/min, hence, one MET equals 3.5 ml O_2/kg/min.[1]

There are two systems in the body for the breakdown of glucose and the production of ATP or energy. One system works in the absence of oxygen and is called anaerobic glycolysis.[6,13,21] This system is inefficient and builds up an inordinate amount of lactic acid which results in a state of acidosis that can lead to early fatigue. Due to the harmful byproducts and a limited amount of available fuel, the body can only function anaerobically for up to a maximum of 40 sec.

The second system is called aerobic glycolysis and functions in conjunction with the Krebs cycle to produce energy.[6,13,21] Oxygen is utilized, in part, to prevent the accumulation of lactic acid. Aerobic glycolysis produces 38 molecules of ATP from one molecule of glucose as compared to two molecules of ATP produced in anaerobic glycolysis. By utilizing the Krebs cycle, aerobic glycolysis becomes a tremendously efficient source of energy that has only ATP, water, and carbon dioxide as its byproducts.[13]

During the stress test, both of these systems come into play.[8] As the warm-up and subsequent stages commence, anaerobic glycolysis supplies the energy required by the increased workload, while the slower responding Krebs cycle increases its production of ATP. As the body begins to function entirely aerobically, it enters a stage called *steady state,*[8] during which time the blood pressure and heart rate should attain constant levels. Steady state is achieved only at lower levels of exertion. At work rates approaching maximum, the Krebs cycle will not be able to completely phase out anaerobic glycolysis. This quickly builds up lactic acid and the body now enters into oxygen debt. The metabolic rate must remain elevated after termination of exercise to pay off or "blow off" this debt. The graph in Figure 2.1 illustrates the interplay of the two energy systems and the resultant condition of oxygen debt.[6,8]

It is possible to predict oxygen consumption ($\dot{V}O_{2\ max}$) from the steady state maximum workload.[10] Indeed, in 1960, Taylor[10] determined "that one can predict oxygen consumption. . . with almost as much accuracy as one can measure it." By using the various formulas and nomagrams available, $\dot{V}O_2$ can be estimated to accuracy which is within acceptable limits. Extensive use has been made of this fact in the determination of functional capacity and exercise prescription.

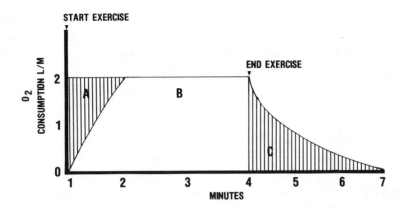

Interplay of aerobic and anaerobic glycolysis. As exercise begins, the initial burst of energy is supplied by anaerobic glycolysis while aerobic glycolysis increases energy production (A). Steady state is attained (B) when all energy is provided through aerobic glycolysis. At the termination of exercise (C), the metabolic rate remains elevated to pay off the accumulated O_2 debt.

During a stress test, the increased demand for oxygen and the byproducts of anaerobic glycolysis are responsible for the changes commonly seen during exertion; i.e., increased heart rate, elevated blood pressure, increased respiratory rate, ST changes, dyspnea, fatigue, claudication and angina pectoris. While all of these changes are physiological responses to exertion, a detailed discussion of their etiology will not be included herein. The reader is referred to the many definitive studies already published on these subjects.

PHYSIOLOGICAL REQUIREMENTS FOR A VALID EXERCISE TOLERANCE TEST

Barnard, et al[22] found that two-thirds of a group of firemen that had previously responded normally to stress tests could be induced to have a marked ischemic response as a result of sudden extreme treadmill exercise that did not allow sufficient time for warm-up. The ischemic response was demonstrated by ST depression which could have caused a false positive diagnosis.

The American College of Sports Medicine, in *Guidelines for Graded Exercise Testing and Exercise Prescription*[1], suggests that a stress test not start at a level in excess of two to three METs. They also suggest that the individual steps not consist of intervals of more than one MET for persons at risk or more than two METs for normal persons. Observation of these suggestions should eliminate the false positive ischemic response due to the onset of extreme workloads and the excess build-up of lactic acid due to failure to attain steady state.[8,22]

The ability to predict VO_2 at various stages of a stress test is essential in tests for diagnosis as well as function. In tests for function the termination of $\dot{V}O_2$ is critical to create an effective exercise prescription, to define the extent of myocardial damage, and to evaluate the efficacy of both medication and conditioning programs.[1,8,16] In diagnostic tests, the level of oxygen consumption at the onset of symptoms can be used to evaluate progress of the disease.

Since it is rare for a patient to actually attain steady state at higher workloads[8], it is imperative that the test intervals not be too extreme in order to allow a closer approximation of $\dot{V}O_{2\ max}$. Although proponents of some protocols have developed regression equations that approximate the $\dot{V}O_2$ at given times in the test, these attempts tend to add even more error to a value which is already difficult to estimate accurately[10]. The stage increments, suggested by the American College of Sports Medicine, of one of two METs per step[1] would tend to decrease some error in $\dot{V}O_2$ prediction. The many protocols in existence should be evaluated to see if they conform to this proposal.

Another practice which adds error to the estimation of $\dot{V}O_2$ is that of allowing the use of the handrail during the test procedure[4,10]. It is impossible to determine the amount of weight being supported by the arms, even if just a finger is used for balance. Studies have shown that as much as three to five minutes can be added to test duration through handrail use.[4] This invalidates the test as far as future reference is concerned, or any determination of aerobic capacity. Out of 300 to 500 stress tests that I have either given or observed in the past year, it has not been necessary for one patient to require the use of the handrail for support or balance, regardless of age or health status. It is wise to allow a short period of time for the patient to become accustomed to the motion of the treadmill. The practice stage should be followed by a short rest before the actual test begins. This effectively eliminates any concern the patient might have regarding his ability to perform the test.

An innovative and important area of stress testing which is gaining more support daily is that of submaximal testing to determine safe functional capacity for post myocardial infarction and cardiac surgery victims prior to release from the hospital. A typical protocol for this procedure would include an initial stage of one MET and subsequent increments of one MET until a heart rate of 120 is reached or contraindications are incurred.

This practice eliminates the uncertainty of releasing high risk patients to go home and "take it easy." Advice can be given on specific levels of activity which will be well tolerated, and medications can be prescribed for any indicated problems. In personal experience with this procedure two out of seven patients tested in a given month incurred life threatening arrhythmias at a level of activity substantially below that normally attained by patients upon their return home.

This procedure, in particular, requires extreme caution in both the design of the test and the conduction thereof. Many patients would need stage increments of one-half MET or less to avoid the problems caused by insufficient warm-up or extreme work-load increases. Again, the people administering the test must know the aerobic principles of stress testing as well as the history of the patient.

Another controversy frequently encountered in stress testing is that of maximum or symptom-limited test vs. submaximal or predetermined endpoint tests. Strong arguments can be made for each of these endpoints. Experience shows, however, that given the many purposes for testing, each manner of determining the endpoint can be useful.

The criteria for stopping a stress test are: exercise limiting fatigue, the emergence of symptoms indicative of cardiac insufficiency, or attainment of a predetermined endpoint, such as 85% of the predicted maximum heart rate. The predetermined endpoint, if sufficiently modified, is the safest for high-risk patients and serves to give the physician useful information on efficacy of medication and activity levels without placing the patient under undue stress.

Regardless of the original purpose for the test, all procedures should be terminated at the onset of symptoms which pose a threat to the patient. This endpoint should be considered maximum for the patient. Many of the patients we have worked with have never attained their true or predicted maximum due to symptoms which cause premature termination. This endpoint still serves as a reference in subsequent tests.

Rochmis and Blackburn[17] have reported that no clear relationship exists between morbidity and mortality and the type of test or intensity of work. Hence, in most cases, the maximum test can be considered as safe as the predetermined endpoint.

Maximum tests have the widest range of use. If not used correctly, however, they can also cause greater error or discrepancy than the other tests. The patient must be encouraged to continue until his fatigue is indeed exercise limiting. If this is not the case, then the data that is accepted as maximal will be very misleading. Cumming found that out of 511 volunteers a full 50% of the ischemic responses would have been missed had the test been terminated at 85% of the predicted maximum heart rate. Hence, for diagnostic value, the maximum stress test must be favored.[1,5,8,16,19]

In tests for function, a maximal test is also the most dependable. The popular formula for estimating one's maximum heart rate is notoriously unreliable: i.e., 220 minus your age.[14,16,19] Blindly following this formula cannot only give unreliable data, but in some cases may even be dangerous to the patient. Although most patients do not reach steady state at maximum workload, a maximal test will still give a better estimation of $\dot{V}O_2$ than will a predetermined endpoint.

It must be emphasized that all of these criteria should be considered to design a protocol which will best suit the aim of the test.

OTHER CONSIDERATIONS IN PROTOCOL DESIGN

Although the treadmill is the recommended instrument for stress testing, there exists as many other mediums for testing as protocols. For the American public the treadmill uses the largest muscle groups resulting in increased stress to the cardiovascular system and is a more reliable test[14,19]. During the procedure, it is relatively simple to get a continuous ECG recording and blood pressure measurement. This type of activity is familiar to all patients, and with the proper precautions is extremely safe. The results are reproducible and an enormous body of knowledge exists concerning possible responses to the test. Depending upon the protocol selected, the duration of the treadmill test is usually negligible.

The positive aspects of treadmill use, as presented above, do not, however, rule out the possible use of other mediums for testing, as in the case of physical limitations or limitations due to budget and space. Bicycle and arm ergometers, single and multi steps, and even timed runs have been employed with lesser degrees of success.[6,8,14,18] Some of these mediums give good results in diagnosis but are unreliable for measurement of functional capacity. The opposite is true for other tests. It is not possible to delve into the strengths and weaknesses of each instrument. Let it suffice to say that the immediate purpose of the test and the limitations of the patient must be considered in selecting the proper method.

Another major consideration in test design is the monitoring and recording devices used. The market is saturated with quality instruments designed to meet the demands of rigorous stress testing. Regardless of the quality of the instrument purchased, the initial preparation must be fastidiously accomplished or the test results will be hopelessly garbled. Needless to say, if the signal received is unintelligible or of no value diagnostically, the test should be stopped immediately.

Without regard to the placement of the skin electrodes, the prep which seems to result in the most consistent tracing consists of: 1) shaving the proposed electrode site, 2) abrading the skin with sandpaper or a burring tool, and 3) cleaning the site with alcohol to remove oil and loose skin. Hair and the horny epidermal layer can obliterate a meaningful signal during exercise and should be removed[8,19]. Personal experience with a small dental burr has produced superior results in the vast majority of patients.

In regards to the placement of the electrodes, Blackburn et al found that 100% of all ischemic responses were seen using leads II, AVF, and V_{3-6}. V_5 is the single most reliable lead to monitor with 89% of all ischemic responses detectable.[3] If modification must be made in a standard protocol, every effort should be made to monitor either all or some combination of these leads.

SUMMARY

The purposes for exercise tolerance testing can be divided into two major categories — diagnostic and functional. To obtain valid results each purpose requires a slow increase in oxygen consumption until a predetermined endpoint or maximum $\dot{V}O_2$ is attained. Care must be taken to prevent the patient from developing a state of acidosis too early in the test or to cause an ischemic response due to insufficient warm-up instead of occlusive disease.

Other factors which must be considered are safety, time, type of activity, equipment required, physical limitations, and purpose of the test. In general, the guidelines for construction and evaluation of an exercise test protocol should include the following requirements as set forth by Ellestad:[8]

1) A type of activity that is relatively familiar or at least within the grasp of the patient.

2) A workload that can be varied according to the capacity of the patient but is sufficiently standardized for at least rough estimates of $\dot{V}O_2$.

3) An activity which lends itself to frequent ECG recordings and blood pressure measurements.

4) Maximum safety and minimum discomfort for the patient.

5) The highest possible sensitivity in the diagnosis of disease.

6) Sufficient information regarding the responses which could be expected during a specific test.

7) Stages of sufficient duration and intensity to allow for warm-up and to attain steady state.

8) Short enough procedure to be practical.

No established protocol has been shown to have a clear-cut advantage over another[10]. The procedure must be adapted both to suit the aim of the test and to allow for the physical limitations of the patient. Knowledge of the aerobic principles of stress testing and an awareness of the strengths and weaknesses of the many procedures and instruments available will aid in the resolution of complications when they arise.

REFERENCES

1. American College of Sports Medicine, Guidelines for Graded Exercise Testing and Exercise Prescription, Great Britain, Lea & Febiger, 1975.

2. American Heart Association, The Committee of Exercise, Exercise Testing and Training of Individuals with Heart Disease or at High Risk for its Development: A Handbook for Physicians, American Heart Association, 1975.

3. Blackburn H, Katigbak R, Mitchell P, Imbimbo B. What electrocardiographic leads to take after exercise? Amer Heart J 67:184-188, 1964. 188, 1964.

4. Copper M, The symptom-limited exercise tolerance test in the diagnosis of coronary artery disease, Cardiology Digest, 10:11-20, 1975.

5. Cumming GR, Yield of ischemic exercise electrocardiograms in relation to exercise intensity in a normal population, Br Heart J, 34:919-923, 1972.

6. DeVries HA, Physiology of Exercise for Physical Education and Activities, Dubuque, Iowa, Wm C Brown Co, 1976, chap 9.

7. Doyle JT, Kinch SH, The prognosis of an abnormal electrocardiographic stress test, Circulation, Vol 61.

8. Ellestad MH, Stress Testing: Principles and Practice, Philadelphia, PA, FA Davis Co, 1975, chaps 2,5,9.

9. Faulkner JA, Heigenhauser GF, Schork MA. The cardiac output — oxygen uptake relationship of men during graded bicycle ergometry, Medicine and Science in Sports, 9:3:148-154, 1977.

10. Froelicher VF, Thompson AJ, Davis F, et al. Prediction of maximal oxygen consumption: comparison of the Bruce and Balke treadmill protocols, Chest, 68:331-336, 1975.

11. Goldschlager N, Cohn K. Treadmill stress tests as indicators of presence and severity of coronary artery disease, Annals of Internal Medicine, 85:3:277-286, 1976.

12. Kattus AA. Exercise electrocardiography: recognition of the ischemic response, false positive and negative patterns, Amer J Cardiol, 33:721-731, 1974.

13. Langley LL, Telford IR, Christensen JB, Dynamic Anatomy & Physiology, New York, McGraw-Hill Book Co, 1974, pp 631-632.

14. McDonough JR, Bruce RA. Maximal exercise testing in assessing cardiovascular function, distributed by Quinton Instruments, Seattle, Washington.

15. National Exercise and Heart Disease Project, Common Protocol, Washington, DC, The George Washington University Medical Center, 1975.

16. Naughton JP, Hellerstein HK. Exercise Testing and Exercise Training in Coronary Heart Disease, New York, Academic Press, Inc, 1973, chaps 4,6.

17. Rochmis P, Blackburn H. Exercise Tests: A survey of procedures, safety and litigation experience in approximately 170,000 tests, JAMA, 19:1, 1976.

18. Schwade J, Shapiro W, Blomquist CG. A comparison of the response to arm and leg work in patients with ischemic heart disease, Amer Heart, 94:203-208, 1977.

19. Scheffield LT, Roitman D. Stress testing methodology, Prog Cardiol, 19:1, 1976.

20. Tanner JM. The construction of normal standards for cardiac output in man, J Clin Inves, 28:567-582, 1949.

21. Vander AJ, Sherman, JH, Luciano DS. Human Physiology: The Mechanics of Body Function, New York, McGraw-Hill Book Co, 1975, pp 78-86.

22. Zohman LR, Kattus AA. Exercise testing in the diagnosis of coronary heart disease: a perspective, Amer J Cardiol, 40:243-249, 1977. 40:243-249, 1977.

A Quantitative Approach to the Noninvasive Diagnosis of Coronary Artery Disease

J. S. Forrester, M.D.
Ran Vas, Ph.D.
G. A. Diamond, M.D.

In the absence of clinical history or findings, the diagnosis of coronary artery disease is quite difficult. Exercise electrocardiography is currently the only widely employed method for the detection of the disease prior to clinical manifestations. Even in the absence of a proven effective therapy, such testing is relevant, since an abnormal test result identifies a group of subjects at a substantially higher risk, in whom preventive measures may be attempted.

The major limitation of this approach, however, is that only about 25% of asymptomatic patients with abnormal ECG exercise tests actually have anatomic disease. The fact that many normal patients are incorrectly placed in a high risk catagory undermines all preventive therapeutic approaches. In the absence of accurate diagnosis, it seems unlikely that even an effective preventive therapeutic approach could be recognized when the vast majority of patients being treated do not, and never will, develop the disease being "treated."

For preventive treatment of asymptomatic diseases, therefore, accurate diagnosis is essential. A number of additional promising noninvasive procedures are available for the more accurate detection of coronary artery disease, but there is no effective format for their serial utilization. The purpose of this discussion is to describe such a format.

THE CONCEPT OF LIKELIHOOD

The format is based on the fact that the results of tests performed may be stated in terms of posttest likelihood for disease. To illustrate how this may be done, assume that in a population of 1000 individuals, 100 have disease, representing a disease prevalence of 10%. Each individual, therefore, has a *pretest likelihood* for disease of 10%. If the ECG stress test were known to have a sensitivity of 70% and a specificity of 90%, the posttest likelihood for disease in an individual with a positive test would be 44%.

If a second, different test were then performed on this individual, the posttest likelihood would again change, depending on the results of the second test. If the latter test had a sensitivity of 60% and a specificity of 80%, then the posttest likelihood would be 70%. Conversely, if the test were negative, the posttest likelihood would be 28%.

35

These examples illustrate how the likelihood for disease may be determined, provided that the sensitivity and specificity of the test and the prevalence (likelihood) of disease in the population is known. With each additional test, two new populations are defined: one with a higher prevalence of disease due to the positive test, the other with a negative result and a lower prevalence of disease. To determine the individual patient's risk, therefore, we will review the available literature concerning disease prevalence and data required for clinical application of the method.

THE PREVALENCE OF CORONARY ARTERY DISEASE

Prevalence of coronary artery disease varies widely in specifically defined patient populations. Table 2.1 summarizes the prevalence of angiographically proven coronary artery disease in 5038 patients defined according to the presence and type of chest pain. Major differences in prevalence of disease are observed in these four populations. In the population with typical angina, the prevalence of coronary disease is approximately 90%, whereas atypical angina has only 50% prevalence. Nonanginal chest pain has a 15% prevalence and the adult population without symptoms has a 5% prevalence of coronary heart disease. These data underscore the value of the clinical history in the diagnosis of coronary artery disease and provide a means for estimating the pretest likelihood in an individual patient.

TABLE 2.1

Angiographic Prevalence Of Coronary Artery Disease By Symptomatic Classification

Symptom	Patients	Prevalence
Typical Angina	1985	89.0 ± 0.7
Atypical Angina	1931	49.9 ± 1.1
Nonanginal chest pain	844	16.0 ± 1.3
Asymptomatic	278	4.5 ± 1.3

Because a positive test in asymptomatic patients still has a low post-test likelihood, it is highly desirable to refine the estimate of pretest likelihood in this population by additional means. The first means for doing so is by age and sex. Table 2.2 summarizes this data in 23,996 autopsied patients. Disease prevalence varies from 0.3% in 30 to 40-year-old females to 12.3% in 60 to 70-year-old males. The mean prevalence in the total population was 4.5%.

TABLE 2.2
Autopsy Prevalence Of Asymptomatic Coronary Artery Disease Classified By Age And Sex

Age	Patients	Prevalence	
		Male	Female
30–40	4499	1.9 ± 0.3	0.3 ± 0.1
40–50	6185	5.5 ± 0.3	1.0 ± 0.2
50–60	6945	9.7 ± 0.4	3.2 ± 0.4
60–70	6367	12.3 ± 0.5	7.5 ± 0.6
Weighted Mean	4.5 ± 0.1		

RISK FACTOR ANALYSIS

A further refinement of the estimate of pretest likelihood is provided, by consideration of certain factors other than age and sex. The Coronary Risk Handbook, distributed by the American Heart Association, provides estimates of coronary artery disease incidence (new disease year) in asymptomatic patients relative to the presence of a number of "risk factors" including smoking history, blood pressure, and serum cholesterol. These data may be converted into prevalence estimates. Table 3.2 shows such derived prevalence data for a 45 to 49-year-old asymptomatic male smoker stratified by the levels of serum cholesterol and systolic arterial pressure. Although the average pretest likelihood for disease in an asymptomatic 45-year-old male is 5.5% according to the autopsy data in Table 2.2, risk factor analysis within this group provides a method whereby pretest likelihood may be estimated to range from 2.9% to 30.5%.

TABLE 2.3

Prevalence of Coronary Artery Disease In A
45 to 49 Year Old Male Smoker*

Cholesterol	SBP 105	120	135	150	165	180	195
185	2.9	3.5	4.2	4.9	6.0	7.1	8.5
210	3.7	4.4	5.4	6.4	7.5	9.0	10.7
235	4.7	5.6	6.7	8.0	9.6	11.4	13.4
260	6.0	7.1	8.4	10.1	12.0	14.2	16.5
285	7.5	8.9	10.6	12.6	14.9	17.4	20.5
310	9.4	11.2	13.3	15.6	18.4	21.6	25.1
335	11.8	14.0	16.5	19.3	22.7	26.4	30.5

* Derived from the Framingham Study (See text)

THE SENSITIVITY AND SPECIFICITY OF DIAGNOSTIC TESTS

Once the pretest likelihood for disease has been determined, it is necessary to know the sensitivity and specificity of the test procedure to determine the posttest likelihood for a given individual. Table 2.4 summarizes these values for commonly available diagnostic tests and test criteria currently in use. In all these data, disease was defined as present or absent by coronary angiography.

The sensitivity of the ECG stress test is largely a function of the magnitude of ST segment depression. Sensitivity inevitably declines as the criterion for a positive test is made more strict, ranging from 65% for > 1.0 mm. depression to 19% for > 2.5 mm. depression. The specificity of the ECG stress test *increases* with more strict criteria, ranging from 85% using the criterion of 1.0 mm. depression to 99% using > 2.5 mm. depression.

Cardiokymography is a new noninvasive technique for recording anterior left ventricular wall motion both at rest and after exercise. In patients

TABLE 2.4
Sensitivity And Specificity Of Noninvasive Tests For Diagnosis Of Coronary Artery Disease

Test	Criterion	Patients	Sensitivity	Specificity
Exercise ECG	0.5 mv	184	85.7 ± 3.3	62.5 ± 5.7
	1.0 mv	4485	64.9 ± 0.9	85.2 ± 0.8
	1.5 mv	785	41.2 ± 2.3	96.3 ± 1.1
	2.0 mv	1157	32.8 ± 1.7	98.3 ± 0.6
	2.5 mv	991	19.6 ± 1.6	99.1 ± 0.5
Fluoroscopy	calcium	485	57.1 ± 2.6	96.4 ± 1.8
Exercise CKG	dyskinesis	227	67.8 ± 4.0	95.6 ± 2.1
Exercise^{201}Tl	hypoperfusion	1134	70.7 ± 1.7	94.0 ± 1.3

with coronary artery disease detection of reversible outward systolic motion induced by treadmill exercise is taken as a positive test response. The sensitivity of the test is 68% and the specificity is 96%.

Perfusion scintigraphy using thallium-201 detects coronary artery disease by means of an exercise-induced prefusion defect not present at rest. The sensitivity of this procedure is 71% and the specificity is 94%.

LIKELIHOOD OF DISEASE FOLLOWING ADDITIONAL TESTS

A 45-year-old asymptomatic male has an average pretest likelihood of 5.5%. If an ECG stress test reveals 1.0 mm. ST segment depression, the posttest likelihood is 20.3%. The use of additional test procedures allows one to define the patient more precisely. Thus, if this patient also had a positive CKG stress test then the posttest likelihood would rise to 80%, and if he also had a positive thallium study, the likelihood for disease would reach 98%. This analysis of likelihood may influence clinical decision making in several ways: First, the quantitative result may indicate a need for further testing, not apparent from the qualitative result alone. For instance, when the posttest likelihood falls into an intermediate range (40% to 60%), additional tests are probably indicated. Conversely, the results may also indicate that further testing would be of little value. For example, if the likelihood was very high (e.g., 95%), little diagnostic gain results from an additional, frequently expensive test. Perhaps most importantly, analysis of likelihood can be used to assess the potential utility of an additional test prior to its actual performance.

These concepts are illustrated in Table 2.5. The hypothetical laboratory report shows the qualitative test results and the calculation of posttest likelihood based upon each result. Beginning with risk factor analysis, the patient has a 2.9% likelihood of having coronary disease. The posttest likelihood after having coronary calcification at fluoroscopy is 35.8%. This is in the intermediate range, in which an ECG stress test would be of value. When the patient exhibits 1.0 mm. ST segment depression after exercise, the likelihood of disease increases to 71.0%. The concordant positive CKG stress test increases this likelihood further to 97.1%. At the bottom, the change in likelihood that would result from performance of a thallium perfusion study is shown for both a positive and negative result. It is seen that a positive perfusion study would only increase likelihood from 97.1% to 99.7%, while a negative study would decrease likelihood only to 91.3%. Thus, with this report, the physician can assess the cumulative effect of multiple, even discordant, test results and evaluate additional procedures prior to their performance. In this example, thallium scintigraphy would appear to add little to the diagnostic evaluation beyond a substantial increase in cost. These calculations of posttest likelihood are within the scope of programmable hand calculators.

TABLE 2.5

| Test | Posttest Likelihood (%) | |
	Negative	Positive
Demographics	2.9	
Fluoroscopy		35.8
ECG Stress		71.0
CKG Stress		97.1
Thallium Stress	91.3	99.7

SUMMARY

Although extensive experience is essential to establish the ultimate clinical relevance of likelihood analysis for diagnosis of ischemic heart disease, this approach holds promise as a method to increase diagnostic accuracy and cost-effectiveness of testing. This format may eventually provide a rational means for the diagnosis of coronary artery disease prior to the appearance of symptoms. Specifically:

1. The accurate interpretation of procedures for diagnosis of ischemic heart disease requires quantitation of three variables: the sensitivity and specificity of the test and the pretest likelihood for disease in the individual being tested. From these data the posttest likelihood for disease may be quantitated according to Bayes' theorem.

2. Pretest likelihood for coronary artery disease may be quantitated in *symptomatic* patients by historical characterization of the various chest pain syndromes, and in *asymptomatic* patients by use of the Coronary Risk Handbook.

3. Quantitation of posttest likelihood when multiple noninvasive test procedures are used follows an identical format to that used in a single test. In each case, the posttest likelihood following one test becomes the pretest likelihood for the next test. This approach to the diagnosis of coronary artery disease may allow its detection prior to the development of symptoms.

REFERENCES

1. McConahay DR, McCallister BD, Smith RE. Post exercise electrocardiography: Correlation with coronary arteriography and left ventricular hemodynamics. Amer J Cardiol. 28: 1, 1972.

2. Proudfit WL, Shirey EK, Sones FM. Selective cine coronary angiography: Correlation with clinical findings in 1000 patients. Circulation 33: 901, 1966.

3. Friesinger GC, Smith RF. Correlation of electrocardiographic studies and arteriographic findings with angina pectoris. Circulation 46: 1173, 1972.

4. Fortuin N.J., Weiss JL. Exercise stress testing. Circulation 56: 699, 1977.

5. Froelicher VF, Thomas MM, Pillow C, et al. Epidemiologic study of asymptomatic men screened by maximal treadmill testing for latent coronary artery disease. Amer J Cardiol 34: 770-776, 1974.

6.   Redwood DR, Borer JS, Epstein SE. Whither the ST segment during exercise? Circulation 54: 703-706, 1976.

7.   Borer JS, Brensike JF, Redwood DR, et al. Limitations of the electrocardiographic response to exercise in predicting coronary artery disease. New Engl J Med 293: 367, 1975.

8.   White NK, Edwards JE, Dry TJ. The relationship of the degree of coronary atherosclerosis with age in men. Circulation 1:645, 1950.

9.   Clawson BJ. Incidence of types of heart disease among 30,265 autopsies with special reference to age and sex. Amer Heart J 17: 607, 1939.

10. Johnston C. Racial difference in the incidence of coronary sclerosis. Amer Heart J

11. Willius FA, Smith HL, Sprague PH. A study of coronary and aortic sclerosis: Incidence and degree in 5060 consecutive postmortem examinations. Proceedings of the Staff Meetings of the Mayo Clinic 8: 140, 1933.

12. Spain DM, Bradess VA, Occupational physical activity and the degree of coronary atherosclerosis in "normal" men. Circulation 22: 239, 1960.

13. Rissanen V, Pyorala K. Coronary and aortic atherosclerosis: A study of a series of violent deaths. Atherosclerosis 19: 221, 1974.

14. Tejada C, Strong JP, Montenegro MR, et al. Distribution of coronary and aortic atherosclerosis by geographic location, race and sex. Laboratory Investigation 18: 509, 1968.

Interpretation of the Exercise Electrocardiogram

Sam A. Kinard, MD, FACC

The treadmill exercise electrocardiogram has gained wide popularity as a useful test in evaluation of patients with heart disease as well as a test for screening patients with suspected coronary arterial disease. The sensitivity and specificity of the test is related in large part to those types of individuals that are being tested. Its sensitivity and specificity can be improved considerably by the addition of other information such as the clinical history, physical examination, known risk factors, as well as the addition of other tests such as myocardial imaging. Its accuracy is also related to the method by which it is performed and the detail given to its interpretation.

A standard twelve-lead electrocardiogram is used to perform the exercise test, and a heart rate of 90% of predicted maximum should be achieved. We use the Bruce protocol, and a positive test is one in which there is 1 mm or greater downsloping or horizontal ST segment depression beyond one minute of recovery, or 1½ mm beyond the J junction immediately after exercise. U-wave inversion in the absence of left ventricular hypertrophy is also considered a positive test. Those things which may interfere with the test are inadequate heart rate response, drugs, (such as digitalis, propranolol, diuretics), the presence of a ventricular conduction defect, electrolyte imbalance, or left ventricular hypertrophy.

The depth of the ST segment depression correlates generally with the severity of coronary arterial disease. Two or 3 mm ST segment depression is associated with an increased incidence of proximal left anterior descending, left main, or triple vessel coronary disease. In general, the extent of coronary arterial disease correlates roughly with the total amount of ST segment depression in all leads but there is much overlap, and therefore one cannot necessarily predict the extent of disease from the sum of the ST segment depression.

The duration of a positive test postexercise would suggest prolonged ischemia and therefore more severe disease, but this is not always helpful in determining the extent of disease.

Those patients who cannot complete stage I have a much higher incidence of coronary disease, triple vessel disease, and left main disease than those who are able to complete stage II. A combination of the depth of ST segment depression equal to or greater than 3 mm, persistence of positivity equal to or greater than 5 min and exercise endurance of less than stage I are always associated with multivessel coronary disease. On the opposite end of the spectrum, those patients who have a negative exercise test, or an exercise duration equal to or greater than stage IV, have a very low incidence of coronary disease.

43

In a recent article, those patients who were able to exercise into stage IV or greater and able to achieve a heart rate of 160 or greater had a 99% 12-month survival and a 95% 48-month survival. Survival in patients stopping exercise at stage I was 85% in 12 months and 78% in 36 months. Of those who achieved a heart rate less than 120 at this level of exercise, survival was 80% at 12 months and 31% in 48 months. Thus, the treadmill exercise test is a strong prognostic indicator.

False positive treadmill tests will occur much more frequently when the treadmill is used as a screening test in asymptomatic individuals. A false positive test is said to be more common in females than in males, and in about half of the patients with false positive tests there are labile ST or T-wave changes that may occur with hyperventilation or after eating and this is the clue to the false positivity. The ST segment depression should continue after the cessation of peak exercise for at least a minute and upsloping ST segment depression should equal 1½ mm 0.08 sec after the J junction.

False negative tests in those patients with significant coronary disease are seen more often in patients with disease of the right or circumflex coronary artery or with single vessel disease and less in those with triple vessel disease or anterior descending disease.

In a patient with a normal resting electrocardiogram, no labile repolarization changes, abnormal ST segment depressions with exercise, and exercise-induced chest pain, there will be significant coronary arterial disease 95% of the time. Conversely, an abnormal stress electrocardiogram in an asymptomatic individual should be considered a risk factor and according to a recent article, there is a 14-fold increase in risk for asymptomatic subjects over a five-or six-year follow-up. The incidence of coronary disease in these individuals is probably about 50%.

The exercise electrocardiogram provides considerably more information than the ST segment changes which may occur. Arrhythmias which may occur only with exercise can be detected and treated appropriately. Although arrhythmias do not mean that the test is positive, one can get an excellent indication of a patient's exercise tolerance and one is able to evaluate the effect of surgical or pharmacological intervention on the exercise tolerance of patients with coronary disease. As a follow-up examination, the treadmill exercise test can provide information regarding deterioration in the patient's exercise ability and stage and heart rate at which ST segment changes occur.

When performed and interpreted properly, and in light of the overall clinical situation, the treadmill exercise test is an invaluable aid in the management of patients with heart disease and is a useful screening test if one recognizes its limitations in this setting.

Section 3

Peripheral and Cerebrovascular Noninvasive Testing

Disorders in the peripheral or cerebrovascular circulation have, until recent times, been diagnosed initially using symptomatology and nonspecific auscultatory or palpable evidence to a large degree. Arteriography of the involved area was the only means of assessing the extent of any condition which may have existed. Although this latter statement is still valid, the preliminary diagnostic procedures have changed drastically.

In response to the need for reliable diagnostic tools for peripheral and cerebrovascular noninvasive testing, research has developed several new techniques which have proven their value as both diagnostic and screening methods. The idea behind the use of these noninvasive tests is the avoidance of unnecessary arteriography and the identification of latent vascular disease. In peripheral vessels, impedance plethysmography and the Doppler ultrasound technique have been used successfully and reliably to assess the level and severity of obstructive lesions and of the veins and arteries, respectively. For the cerebrovascular system, oculoplethysmography and carotid phonoangiography form a tandem testing protocol to localize and quantify stenotic lesions in the carotid circulation.

The papers on these noninvasive testing procedures explain their use, interpretation, diagnostic significance, and reliability. Moreover, insight is offered into the developments, both present and future, which will affect the usefulness of these diagnostic tools.

Bi-Directional Doppler:
Technical Considerations in Testing

Marilyn Reiling, RN, CVS, RT, BS

Peripheral vascular disease poses a major threat to the American people, and is more prevalent than coronary artery disease. Coronary and vascular diseases represent the single greatest cause of death in the United States today. Peripheral vascular disease does not have a high percentage of mortality. However, it does have economic losses from work due to inability to ambulate, socialization losses from inactivity, and loss of well being from impotency.

The nurse's primary role in this topic is to enhance evaluation of peripheral vascular disease. Presently, nurses are expected to review neurological, cardiac, renal, and other systems of the body in their nursing history evaluation, as well as day-to-day evaluation in nurses' notes and progress reports. Palpating pulses are not reliable in the presence of decreased cardiac output, vasoconstricting medication, and cold feet. Evaluation of the peripheral vascular system by Doppler ultrasound has been introduced and found to be safe, effective, reliable and painless.

Christian Doppler discovered the Doppler effect in 1842, and he theorized "the frequency of sound waves when emitted or reflected from a moving object varies in proportion to the velocity of the object relative to the observer."[1] To simplify this for our purposes, moving blood cells in sufficient number reflect high-frequency ultrasound. The reflection of this frequency is the "Doppler shift." The Doppler shift can be used to detect velocity of blood flow and systolic pressures in the leg.

The Doppler instrument is primarily an electronic device which has a hand-held probe with a crystal in the probe. This crystal vibrates when fed electrical energy to generate high frequency ultrasound. The hand-held probe can be obtained to vary in frequency from 5 to 8 MHz for peripheral vascular evaluation. The lower megahertz has a deeper penetration and less resolution, with the higher megahertz having better resolution with less penetration. The 5 MHz probe works very well for venous detection because it has penetration of 2 to 3 in. The 8 MHz probe works very well for arterial detection because it has a depth of 1 to 1.5 in. and good resolution for distinct audible and wave tracing recordings.

The piezoelectric crystal within the hand-held probe receives electrical energy and converts the energy to high frequency ultrasound. The high frequency ultrasound cannot be heard by the human ear. There are two crystals in the hand-held probe: the transmitting crystal from which the ultrasound leaves the probe, and the receiving crystal which assesses the "Doppler shift" from returning ultrasound. Energy reflected from stationary boundaries is received back at the original transmitted frequency, while energy reflected from moving boundaries suffers a change in frequency proportional to the velocity of the boundaries.[2] Soft tissues and fluids absorb little ultrasound. So ultrasound which passes through hard tissue such as bone absorbs high frequency ultrasound and causes extensive scattering which does not come back to the receiving crystal and therefore cannot be measured. Moving fluid reflects the ultrasound and this is detected by the receiving crystal with a change in frequency proportional to the velocity of the blood.

Technique in using the Doppler instrument can be easily learned. Ultrasound does not travel well through air, and therefore coupling gel must be used between the probe and the skin. The transmitting and receiving crystal have an angle which can vary slightly in different instruments. To obtain maximum Doppler shift the angle of the probe should be 45° to the vessel being examined. This does not mean 45° to the skin. Occasionally, when listening to popliteal and femoral arteries, the probe is at a 90° angle to the skin to obtain a 45° angle to the artery.

Finding the optimum 45° angle will come with experience and exploration of different arteries. A directional Doppler component with stereo headsets will separate advancing flow in one ear and receding flow in the other ear. The probe can therefore be positioned to obtain arterial flow in one ear and venous flow in the other ear. A directional Doppler is informative and helpful in recording tracings. It is not necessary in evaluating pressures and therefore this discussion will include only a nondirectional Doppler (sound heard equally in both ears). Most pocket sized Dopplers used at the bedside are nondirectional Dopplers.

Peripheral vascular disease compromises blood flow to the extremities which results in pain, ulceration and tissue death. Factors influencing blood flow are pressure, blood volume and resistance. To maintain common terminology, these factors will be defined:

Blood Flow - Quantity of blood flowing through a vessel at a given period of time.

Velocity - Distance that blood travels along a vessel in a given period of time.

Pressure - Amount of force exerted against the walls of the artery.

Resistance - Friction between blood and the vessel wall that creates impedance to flow. Resistance is dependent on length of vessel, diameter of vessel and viscosity of blood.

The body is very complex in regulating blood flow. Listed below are some factors that affect blood flow.[3]

Pressure	Volume	Resistance
1. Baroreceptors at carotid bifurcation and aorta increase pressure	Kidneys regulate blood volume by responding to pressure and flow going through the kidney	Changes in diameter of vessel such as vaso-constriction and vaso-dilitation
2. Vasomotor in brain decreases pressure and works with barorecep-tors to keep pressure in balance	Aldosterone — descreases kidney output of sodium chloride and water	Irregularities such as openings or blockage of vessels
3. Renin — Angiotensin increases pressure	Capillary fluid exchange regulates volume level	Increased viscosity of blood
4. Metabolities of CO_2 and lactic acid during increase pressure	Nervous system regulates heart rate which can affect blood volume	
5. Ischemia increases pressure		

With these many variables, it may appear that studying the pressure could be very difficult. There are, however, some laws of blood flow which help in assessing the pressure-flow relationship. Poiseuille's Law:

$$\text{Blood Flow} = \frac{\text{Pressure} \times \text{Diameter}^4}{\text{Length} \times \text{Viscosity}}$$

In this formula, pressure and blood flow velocity will be used to assess blood flow. This will begin with the discussion of pressure.

The pressure in the ankle should be equal to or greater than the pressure in the arm. If the pressure in the ankle is lower than the arm, the blood flow is being compromised to the extremity. The reason why the pressure is not lost or decreased in the ankle under normal conditions is that there is little pressure loss in the arteries themselves. Most of the pressure is lost past the arteries. To be more specific, one half of the pressure is lost at the arterioles and one fourth is lost at the capillar level.

Example: Mean pressure at various levels

Aorta   100 mm Hg.

Arteries   85 mm Hg.

Arterioles   55 mm Hg.

Capillaries   30 mm Hg.

End Capillaries   10 mm Hg.[4]

Therefore, the arteries, whether arm or leg, will be equivalent. The reason why the ankle is slightly higher has been theorized that there is less resistance in distal vessels and gravity may have an effect of increased pressure in the ankle. For sure there is no reason for the pressure in the ankle to be lower than the arm.

To use this principle of pressure, the ankle pressure must equal the arm pressure and if the ankle pressure is lower, the blood flow is being compromised to the extremity. A grading system has been worked out to assist in evaluating the degree of blood flow compromise. The grading system utilizes a ratio of the ankle pressure divided by the arm pressure.

Example:

$$\frac{\text{Ankle Systolic Pressure}}{\text{Arm Systolic Pressure}} = \text{ratio}$$

The grading system is as follows:

1.00-above   = Normal to minimal disease

.70-.99   = Moderate disease

.69-below   = Significant arterial disease

The following is a basic procedure for recording ankle/arm systolic Doppler pressures:

1. Patient must be lying flat or with a pillow.

2. No exercise should be done for 20 min prior to recording pressures.

3. Standard size arm blood pressure cuff is used for arm and ankle pressures.

4. Coupling gel is placed on the skin over the area of the artery.

5. A maximum signal is obtained by holding probe at 45° angle to the artery.

6. Obtain a clear signal and inflate the blood pressure cuff approximately 20 mm Hg above the level at which the Doppler sounds stop.

7. Slowly deflate the cuff until the first audible Doppler sound is heard. This is the systolic pressure. There is no diastolic pressure with this method because the Doppler signal is heard equally throughout once systole is heard. The systolic pressure is all that is necessary in computing the ankle/arm ratio.

8. Record both arm systolic pressures and use the highest pressure for computing the ratio.

9. The same size cuff should be used for the ankle pressures as used for the arm pressures so comparable values are obtained.

10. Apply the blood pressure cuff just above the ankle.

11. To obtain the ankle systolic pressure, locate the posterior tibial artery which is just below the medial malleolus. The posterior tibial artery usually has the highest pressure in the ankle. The highest pressure is needed to compute the ankle/arm ratio. If unable to use the posterior tibial artery, use the dorsalis pedis artery on the top of the foot, and if unable to use the dorsalis pedis artery, then use the Peroneal artery on the lateral aspect of the foot.

Consideration will now be given to velocity. Velocity is the audible part of the Doppler signal. It is important to understand the audible signal to be sure the listener is over an artery and not a vein. The pressure in a vein will be 45 mm Hg and this, if computed into a ratio, would clearly indicate an abnormal ankle/arm ratio.

There are, however, many instances when the arterial leg pressure is 45 mm Hg and below, and therefore one cannot assume a low pressure is a venous pressure.

Components of the Doppler Signal

Arterial	Venous
Pulsatile	Varies with respirations
Systolic and diastolic components	Sounds like a wind storm
Squeeze distal part, (e.g., squeeze foot if listening to ankle) sound remains the same	Squeeze distal part, sound increases

It is important to follow these guidelines because a diseased artery can sometimes sound like a vein and distal squeezing will distinguish the artery from the vein.

Peripheral vascular disease deserves evaluation because of the serious nature of this progressive disease. Recording ankle/arm Doppler systolic pressures at the bedside to determine the presence of significant arterial disease can be easily done. Progress in early detection and prevention of peripheral vascular disease is only as good as our contribution as concerned medical personnel.

REFERENCES

1.   Versatone-Medsonics Pamphlet, Mountain View, CA, Jan 1976, p 3.

2.   MJ Teague, Sonicaid Pamphlet, Sonicaid Bognor Regis, West Sussex, England, 1976, p 6.

3.   Function of the Human Body, 4th Edition, AC Guyton Ed., WB Saunders Co, Philadelphia, 1974, pp 132-138.

4.   Ibid., p 131.

Challenges in Interpretation of Noninvasive Tests of Peripheral Arterial Disease

Robert W. Barnes, MD

Until recently, the evaluation of peripheral arterial disease has involved the three basic steps of history, physical examination and arteriography. While such techniques remain the cornerstones for patient management, the past decade has witnessed increasing use of noninvasive diagnostic testing to detect, localize and quantify arterial occlusive disease. Such techniques have permitted repeated physiological testing of the patient without risk or discomfort to the individual. With the rapid emergence of noninvasive vascular laboratory techniques, problems have arisen in several areas, including confusion about what techniques are to be preferred, misunderstanding of the principles and applications of the modalities, and misinterpretations of the role of noninvasive testing in the total evaluation and therapy of the patient. The purpose of this paper is to review the practical noninvasive techniques that are currently available and to outline the principles, applications and interpretations of the various modalities of patient evaluation. An understanding of these principles is important not only to the physician responsible for the patient, but also to the nurse, technician or other paramedical person who carries out the noninvasive vascular laboratory tests.

TECHNIQUES

There are two basic techniques which have found practical application in the noninvasive peripheral vascular laboratory: Doppler ultrasound and plethysmography. The following section will review the principles of these two instruments and will outline the basic methods that can be carried out with these devices.

DOPPLER ULTRASOUND

Principles. The Doppler ultrasonic velocity detector consists of a hand-held probe which emits a beam of ultrasound into the tissues through an acoustic gel coupling with the skin. Sound reflected from moving blood cells is shifted in frequency and detected and amplified by the instrument as an audible signal or a recordable analogue waveform.

Instrumentation. Doppler ultrasonic devices may use either continuous or pulse-wave techniques. Most commercially-available instruments for use in the peripheral vascular laboratory are continuous-wave devices. Pulsed instruments are especially useful in research or for noninvasive imaging of arteries (ultrasonic arteriograph). The Doppler devices may be nondirectional, which are less expensive, or may have direction-sensing capability. The latter instruments are particularly useful for recording arterial velocity waveforms in peripheral arterial or cerebrovascular evaluation.

Methods. The two most useful techniques to evaluate peripheral arterial disease by Doppler ultrasound are:

1.   Velocity signal analysis
2.   Limb blood pressure measurement

Velocity signals may be assessed audibly or may be visually analyzed from recorded waveforms. Normally the peripheral arterial velocity signal is multiphasic with a prominent systolic component and one or more diastolic sounds. The arterial signal distal to an arterial obstruction is attenuated with a less prominent systolic component and loss of normal diastolic sounds. In advanced arterial occlusive disease with poor collateral circulation, the arterial velocity signal may not be detectable. Limb systolic blood pressure measurements are determined by using the Doppler detector as a sensitive electronic stethoscope. The systolic pressure at any site on the limb is determined by noting the point at which the distal arterial velocity signal returns after deflating a pneumatic cuff from suprasystolic pressures. Normally segmental limb blood pressures are determined at the proximal thigh, above-knee, below-knee and ankle levels. In addition, digit blood pressures are important particularly in diabetes or advanced arterial occlusive disease. The Doppler detector may permit detection of blood flow in the digits, although with advanced arterial disease, digit blood pressures may require plethysmography for measurement. A final application of Doppler ultrasound in peripheral arterial disease is the noninvasive imaging of arteries using the ultrasonic arteriograph.

PLETHYSMOGRAPHY

Principles. Plethysmography refers to the recording of changes in digit or limb dimension with each heart beat or in response to temporary obstruction of venous return with a pneumatic cuff (venous occlusion plethysmography).

Instrumentation. A variety of plethysmographic transducers are available, including water (ocular plethysmograph, OPG); air (pulse volume recorder, PVR; oculo-pneumoplethysmograph, OPG; and phleborheograph, PRG); mercury strain-gauge (Whitney, SPG); impedance (IPG); or photoelectric (PPG) techniques. The author has preferred the mercury strain-gauge and photoplethysmographic techniques because of their simplicity and low cost.

Methods. The various types of plethysmographs permit physiologic assessment of the peripheral circulation by one of the following four basic techniques.

1. Pulse waveform analysis
2. Pulse amplitude quantification
3. Pulse wave transmission or arrival time
4. Limb blood flow quantification by venous occlusion plethymography

Visual inspection of pulse wave contour permits a differentiation of normal pulses, which have steep upslopes, a relatively sharp peak and a dicrotic wave on the downslope, from abnormal pulses which are attenuated, with a more gradual upslope, a rounded peak and loss of the dicrotic wave. A unique type of pulse is characteristic of Raynaud's syndromes, with a "peaked pulse" which characteristically has an anacrotic notch on the upslope, a sharp peak, and a high position of the dicrotic wave on the downslope.

Pulse amplitude quantification permits documentation of attenuation of pulse height with increasing arterial occlusive disease or in response to compression maneuvers of the artery supplying the region being monitored (supra-orbital photoplethysmography). An increase in pulse amplitude is normally present in response to a period of reactive hyperemia following temporary limb ischemia induced by a tourniquet. Absence of reactive hyperemia is evidence of maximal vasodilation of the digit or extremity. Normally pulse amplitude is diminished in response to a deep breath, a reflection of a sympathetic-mediated reflex. Absence of such plethysmographic pulse attentuation in response to a deep breath is indirect evidence of absence of sympathetic vasomotor tone, a situation often present in diabetic extremities. The pulse wave transmission may be delayed in the presence of arterial occlusive disease and is the basis for the detection of extracranial carotid artery occlusive disease with the ocular phethysmograph (OPG).

Finally, the most accurate way to quantify limb blood flow noninvasively is the measurement of arterial flow by venous occlusion plethysmography. The rate of increase in limb volume in response to temporary obstruction of venous return is directly proportional to the rate of arterial blood flow, which may be measured in cc/min/100 gm of tissue. In addition, venous occlusion plethysmography permits determination of maximum venous outflow from the rate of decrease in limb volume following deflation of a venous occlusive cuff. This technique permits accurate noninvasive detection of deep vein thrombosis.

APPLICATIONS AND INTERPRETATIONS

There are five basic applications of the noninvasive peripheral vascular laboratory in patients with suspected peripheral arterial occlusive disease:

1. Objective confirmation of diagnosis
2. Quantification of physiologic impairment
3. Prediction of therapeutic results
4. Monitoring of therapy
5. Following the course of disease

OBJECTIVE CONFIRMATION OF DIAGNOSIS

The history remains the most important method of evaluating patients with suspected peripheral arterial occlusive disease. However, many patients have ambiguous symptoms and other patients may have arterial disease without clinical manifestations. The noninvasive laboratory is useful to objectively detect the presence and location of peripheral arterial disease.

Chronic Arterial Occlusive Disease. Most noninvasive vascular laboratory studies are directed at patients with chronic arterial occlusive disease, usually secondary to atherosclerosis. Such patients usually present to the clinician with claudication (muscular pain brought on by exercise and relieved by rest), rest pain (pain in the foot or toes, especially at night, associated with advanced arterial occlusive disease) or tissue necrosis (ischemic ulceration or gangrene). The presence of chronic arterial occlusive disease can be established by the determination of abnormal distal arterial velocity signals and the presence of an abnormal ankle blood pressure relative to that of the arm (ankle/arm pressure index, API, normally equal to or greater than 1.0). In the presence of arterial occlusive disease the ankle pressure will be below that of the arm by an amount proportional to the degree of circulatory impairment. Patients with claudication may have an API between 0.5 and 1.0. Patients with rest pain or tissue necrosis usually have an API less than 0.5, with an absolute ankle pressure usually less than 50 mm Hg. Localization of the arterial occlusive disease in the leg is possible by measuring segmental leg pressures at the proximal thigh, above-knee, below-knee and ankle levels. Aorto-iliac disease results in a low proximal thigh pressure; femoro-popliteal disease results in a low above-knee or below-knee pressure; and tibio-peroneal disease (especially in diabetics) results in an abnormal pressure gradient between the below-knee and ankle cuffs. Diabetics also may have abnormal pressure gradients between the ankle and the toe.

Normally the systolic pressure gradients between adjacent levels on the limb should be no greater than 30 mm Hg, with greater pressure drops signifying arterial occlusive disease between the sites of measurement. The status of the peripheral vasomotor tone can be assessed by digit photoplethysmography (or other plethysmographic techniques). With progressive arterial occlusive disease, there is proportional vasodilation of the peripheral extremity in order to maintain normal resting blood flow. This phenomenon may be documented by noting attenuation or absence of increased digit pulse amplitudes during reactive hyperemia following temporary foot ischemia. Lack of any increased digit pulse amplitude during reactive hyperemia signifies maximal vasodilation, which occurs in advanced arterial occlusive disease. Such situations preclude benefit from lumbar sympathectomy. Foot sympathetic tone may also be assessed by noting the response of digit pulse amplitude to a deep breath. Absence of any attenuation of digit pulse amplitude signifies loss of sympathetic innervation, a particularly common situation in the diabetic patient.

Acute Arterial Occlusive Disease. Screening techniques similar to that mentioned above may be used in the patient with acute arterial occlusive disease. Such disease may occur as a result of thrombosis superimposed upon underlying atherosclerosis or as a consequence of embolism, particularly from cardiac disease. In addition, these noninvasive techniques permit rapid detection and quantification of arterial injury associated with trauma. A particular type of iatrogenic trauma is the arterial obstruction which may occur following cardiac catheterization or the use of indwelling arterial monitoring catheters. Such arterial occlusive disease is often asymptomatic and unrecognized unless sensitive noninvasive techniques are used, such as Doppler ultrasound. The disease may be prospectively identified by noting the presence of abnormal arterial velocity signals or reduced segmental pressures distal to the site of arterial catheterization.

Ambiguous Symptoms. Noninvasive techniques provide objective validation of the presence or absence of arterial occlusive disease in patients with atypical symptoms, such as pseudoclaudication associated with neuromuscular disease or leg cramps that may mimic vascular rest pain.

Raynaud's Syndromes. Patients with cold sensitivity may be evaluated by Doppler ultrasonic assessment of arterial velocity signals and digit blood pressures. Low digit blood pressures suggest organic occlusive disease (Raynaud's phenomenon) while vasospasm in the absence of arterial occlusive disease should not result in loss of arterial signals or abnormally low digit blood pressures (Raynaud's disease). In addition, abnormal plethysmographic pulse waveforms (peaked pulse) may be further objective evidence of episodic digital ischemia.

Thoracic Outlet Compression. The digit photoplethysmograph is useful to monitor the digit circulation during various maneuvers (Adson, costoclavicular, and hyperabduction) to assess thoracic outlet compression as a cause of upper extremity pain or ischemia.

Arteriovenous Fistula. The abnormal hemodynamics associated with an arteriovenous fistula may be assessed by both Doppler ultrasound and plethysmography. Doppler ultrasound permits assessment of increased arterial flow velocity in the feeding artery and the abnormal signals and pressure gradients distal to the fistula. Plethysmography permits quantification of abnormal blood flow in such conditions.

Compartment Compression. The use of Doppler ultrasound permits assessment of abnormally elevated muscle compartment pressure associated with trauma or circumferential burns. Although direct muscle pressure measurements or compartment blood flow determinations (by Xenon washout) may be necessary to accurately determine compartment compression syndromes, abnormal arterial velocity signals proximal or distal to the compartment in question may suggest compartment compression.

Screening Techniques. Noninvasive laboratory studies permit rapid screening of "high-risk" or asymptomatic patients for subclinical peripheral arterial disease. Patients with diabetes, hyperlipidemia, hypertension, coronary artery disease and other risk factors for atherosclerosis may be appropriately screened for peripheral arterial occlusive disease using Doppler ultrasound and/or plethysmography.

QUANTIFY PHYSIOLOGICAL IMPAIRMENT

The resting determinations of peripheral arterial velocity signals, ankle and segmental leg pressures and digit or limb plethysmographic waveforms provide evidence of the presence and relative magnitude of peripheral arterial occlusive disease. However, the best functional test of the circulation to response to stress is the performance of a hyperemia test. There are two basic types of hyperemia: 1) postexercise, and 2) postischemic (reactive).

Postexercise Hyperemia. The standard technique of measuring the hemodynamic response to stress is the determination of the ankle pressure response to a period of treadmill exercise. A standard method is to have the patient walk at 2 mph on a 12% grade for 5 min or until the patient is forced to stop because of claudication. The ankle pressures are measured in the immediate postexercise period and compared with preexercise values. Normally the ankle pressure will not fall following such exercise. In the presence of arterial occlusive disease the ankle pressure will fall by an amount and duration proportional to the degree of circulatory impairment. The ankle pressure may not rise to the preexercise value for as long as 20 to 30 min following exercise in patients with arterial occlusive disease.

Reactive (Postischemic) Hyperemia. Another technique of stressing the limb arterial circulation is to render the extremity temporarily ischemic (3 to 5 min) with an arterial tourniquet inflated above the systolic blood pressure. Following deflation of the tourniquet the ankle pressure may be repeatedly measured (every 15 sec) during the ensuing period of reactive hyperemia. Normally such hyperemia results in a transient (less than 60 sec) fall in ankle pressure which should not drop below 65% of the preischemic value. A greater drop in ankle pressure for a longer duration reflects arterial occlusive disease and is proportional to the severity of the obstruction. An advantage of reactive hyperemia is the fact that the method requires no special equipment and can be carried out on patients who are unable to walk on a treadmill (amputees, debilitated individuals). In addition, the period of reactive hyperemia is relatively short and conserves the time of a laboratory technician.

PREDICTION OF THERAPEUTIC RESULTS

A unique attribute of the noninvasive peripheral vascular laboratory is the ability to predict whether or not a given surgical procedure will result in significant relief of the patient's symptoms. We have used the laboratory data to predict the efficacy of surgical therapy on the following four conditions:

1. Aorto-iliac reconstruction
2. Femoro-popliteal bypass
3. Lumbar sympathectomy
4. Amputation

Aorto-iliac Reconstruction. Patients with isolated aorto-iliac occlusive disease are relieved by aorto-iliac endarterectomy or aorto-femoral bypass. However, patients with multisegmental arterial occlusive disease may or may not be benefited by an isolated aorto-iliac reconstructive procedure. In general only approximately 70% or 80% of patients are significantly improved by such a procedure. We have found that the noninvasive laboratory provides predictive clues as to which patients will be insufficiently improved following isolated aorto-iliac reconstruction for multisegmental arterial occlusive disease. Patients who fail to gain significant improvement usually have a higher proximal thigh pressure (greater than 85% of the arm systolic pressure), and such patients usually have two or more abnormal pressure gradients in the leg.

Femoro-popliteal Bypass. Patients undergoing femoro-popliteal bypass must be assessed for adequacy of arterial inflow as well as adequacy of arterial outflow. Patients who fail to benefit from a femoro-popliteal bypass usually have many abnormal pressure gradients in the leg and an ankle pressure index of less than 0.2 However, all patients with threatened limb loss should be evaluated by arteriography to determine if arterial reconstruction is feasible. Some patients may have poor visualization of the distal runoff in the leg at the time of arteriography. However, if an arterial velocity signal is audible at the ankle by Doppler ultrasound, that vessel usually is patent and may be considered for arterial reconstruction.

Lumbar Sympathectomy. Patients with advanced arterial occlusive disease are often recommended for lumbar sympathectomy. However less than one-half of such patients will benefit from this procedure. Lumbar sympathectomy is of no value in the relief of claudication. Some patients with early foot ischemia may be relieved by a sympathectomy. The noninvasive laboratory is useful to predict the benefit of such a procedure. Patients who demonstrate intact sympathetic vasomotor tone by vasoconstriction during a deep breath (digit plethysmography) may be helped by a sympathectomy. The best test of the capacity of the peripheral circulation to dilate is the determination of increased digit pulse amplitude in response to reactive hyperemia. If no augmentation of pulse amplitude occurs during such a procedure, the patient is maximally vasodilated and will not be benefited by lumbar sympathectomy.

Amputation. Amputation for advanced arterial occlusive disease must be considered as a useful measure to aid in rehabilitation. The objective of amputation in such patients is to achieve preservation of maximal limb length as well as limb function. In general the amputation should attempt to preserve the knee joint, and if possible to preserve the foot (digit or transmetatarsal amputation).

With advanced arterial occlusive disease such distal amputations may fail to heal. The noninvasive laboratory is useful to predict the level of successful healing of an amputation. In general amputation of the digits or foot will fail to heal if the ankle or toe pressure is less than 50 mm Hg. In diabetic patients the pressure must be 70 mm Hg or greater for such a distal amputation to heal. A below-knee amputation is doomed to failure if no below-knee pressure is detectable and if no arterial signal is audible in the popliteal fossa. Patients with a detectable below-knee pressure of 70 mm Hg or less may or may not heal, but an amputation to preserve the knee joint is recommended. Patients with a below-knee pressure greater than 70 mm Hg almost always will heal, even if wound breakdown occurs and secondary healing is required.

60

MONITORING OF THERAPY

The noninvasive techniques are useful to assess the integrity of arterial reconstructions at the time of operation. In general two types of measurements are obtained in the operation room:

1. Measurement of ankle blood pressures.
2. Doppler assessment of arterial blood flow velocity.

Pressure Measurements. Measurement of ankle systolic blood pressure as compared to the arm (ankle pressure index) is useful to assess the success of aorto-iliac reconstruction, femoral endarterectomy or profundaplasty. Ankle cuffs are placed at the time of induction of anesthesia and ankle/arm pressure index is determined after the patient is anesthetized. Following the completion of the operative procedure, an ankle pressure index is again determined in order to detect the presence of operative complications and assess the efficacy of the reconstructive procedure. The ankle pressure index should increase by at least 10% if the patient is to benefit from the operative procedure. Lesser degrees of improvement or worsening of the ankle pressure index is an indication to perform an arteriogram to detect an arterial thrombosis or embolus. If such a lesion is not found, the patient should be considered for additional distal reconstructive procedures to avoid the necessity of a second operative procedure in the very early postoperative period.

Arterial Velocity Signals. Patients undergoing carotid endarterectomy, femoro-popliteal bypass and renal or mesenteric arterial reconstruction may be assessed for arterial flow velocity signals at the reconstructed segments. A sterile Doppler probe is used to detect the character of the arterial velocity signal in the afferent and efferent arterial segments. The normal velocity signal is multiphasic with prominent flow velocity in diastole. In the presence of an arterial stenosis the arterial signal is high-pitched and turbulent and the signal distal to the arterial obstruction is attenuated with loss of the normal diastolic sounds.

FOLLOWUP OF COURSES OF DISEASE

The objective noninvasive diagnostic techniques mentioned above are very useful to detect the natural history of arterial disease or the influence of medical or surgical therapy. In general, the simplest technique is to measure the ankle/arm pressure index to diagnose arterial disease and judge its magnitude. Patients with claudication may be followed by periodic exercise tests. Some patients may develop a deterioration of limb hemodynamics prior to the development of symptoms and such individuals are candidates for possible

61

arteriography and arterial reconstruction prior to failure of an operative bypass graft. Patients who undergo arterial reconstruction may be assessed prior to discharge from the hospital. If the ankle pressure index is not increased by at least 10% over the preoperative value, a successful result from the operation is unlikely.

CONCLUSIONS

Noninvasive peripheral vascular screening techniques are simple, safe, rapid and accurate reflections of the status of the peripheral circulation in patients with arterial occlusive disease. Such tests may be repeatedly performed by an experienced technician and the resulting physiological information provides useful data about the presence, location, magnitude and course of arterial occlusive disease. Such noninvasive information must be considered an objective complement to the data obtained from the history, physical examination and arteriogram of such patients. It is important to realize that noninvasive diagnostic techniques may be performed by dedicated nurses, technicians or other paramedical personnel who are trained and experienced in such procedures. Such information may not only complement conventional diagnostic procedures, but may increase the diagnostic acumen of physicians caring for patients with peripheral arterial occlusive disease.

Oculoplethysmography and Carotid Phonoangiography — A Noninvasive Procedure for the Prevention of Stroke

Valerie Crain, RN, BSN

The sudden onset of a severe, focal central neurological deficit usually consisting of weakness or paralysis has, by common usage of both physicians and laymen, been labeled as a stroke. The use of this term has usually implied that the neurological deficit is of vascular origin and will be implied in this paper as well.

There are three basic types of strokes — the embolic, ischemic, and hemorrhagic — with controversial percentages associated with each type. [4,18,3] Generally, each type is responsible for approximately one-third of all the frank strokes.

Cerebrovascular accidents (CVA's) are often preceded by transient ischemic attacks (TIA's). A TIA is a focal dysfunction which returns to its predysfunction state within 24 hours. A well respected symptom usually associated with this disease phenomenon is amourosis fugax — a temporary blindness of one eye.

A patient who has a TIA signalling an impending stroke will generally undergo arteriography. Arteriography has long been, and remains, the definitive diagnostic maneuver to determine the degree and localization of stenotic or ulcerative carotid disease. Carotid arteriography has become progressively safer. However, it still poses certain hazards as well as considerable expense to the patient.

When arteriography indicates a plaque or blockage at a surgically accessible site, and the associated clinical symptoms are observed, the patient will be scheduled for a carotid endarterectomy. This surgical procedure is relatively new and was first reported in 1956. The stroke mortality rate associated with this procedure varies from 1% to 21% in different centers. [6,5,18] Many strokes, however, are not preceded by these mild warning symptoms, or the symptoms are ignored. The risk factor of carotid endarterectomy during an evolving stroke is so high that surgery is generally deferred.

A completed stroke is a serious and incapacitating disorder with incalculable social and economic consequences to the patient and his family. Many dollars are spent each year for rehabilitation and although there are many new advances in the field of rehabilitation, the damage is usually permanent and the patient is left with varying degrees of neurological deficit.

Because of the associated risk of arteriography and surgery, along with the social and economic impact stroke has on society, noninvasive studies are essential to prevent needless arteriograms and surgery, and hopefully, to prevent a completed stroke. Noninvasive studies for prevention of stroke provide a new field of technology and diagnostics which is being added to the medical forefront throughout the country in major hospitals as well as in private offices.

HISTORICAL

A brief historical overview of the noninvasive procedures relating to cerebral vascular disease indicates that possibly the earliest and still very effective noninvasive diagnostic test is that of auscultation for carotid bruits using the stethoscope.[9] The effectiveness of this noninvasive test is very dependent upon the skill and experience of the person listening for the bruit. Carotid phonoangiography was developed in an effort to add objectivity to this noninvasive test.

The noninvasive diagnostic test with the second greatest historical impact in carotid occlusive disease is ophthalmodynamometry (ODM).[17] In the hands of a skilled practitioner ODM is effective in detecting acute severe carotid occlusive disease; but a patient with a positive test will often revert to a negative test as collateral circulation develops. Nevertheless, ophthalmodynamometry has served as the inspiration for other noninvasive diagnostic tests including carotid compression tonography,[2] suction ophthalmodynamometry,[7] oculopneumoplethysmography,[8] and oculoplethysmography.[12] The latter of these techniques will be the primary subject of this paper.

The various tests using the eye to detect carotid occlusive disease depend on the ophthalmic artery as the first primary branch of the internal carotid artery. However, other noninvasive studies focus on the supraorbital or frontal circulation as an extension of the ophthalmic artery. Noninvasive carotid occlusive disease evaluations resulting from this line of investigation include frontal thermography,[16,10] supraorbital plethysmography,[1] and supraorbital artery Doppler evaluations.[1,14]

With the rapid development of Doppler and ultrasonic imaging techniques, there is great promise for noninvasive imaging of the carotid system providing graphic representations similar to those which are now obtained only by invasive carotid arteriography.

METHOD

Oculoplethysmography (OPG) and carotid phonoangiography (CPA) are two complementary noninvasive tests for detecting stenotic or occlusive lesions in the carotid system. These tests are now being utilized in many non-invasive laboratories for patients when cerebrovascular symptoms or the risk factors suggest possible impending stroke. Common risk factors include hypertension, diabetes, other known vascular or cardiac disease, and family history of cardiovascular disease. The tests can be used not only for the workup of hospital patients but also as part of the yearly physical as an outpatient.

Oculoplethysmography uses the comparative timing of simultaneously recorded bilateral ocular pulse waveforms. These pulses are obtained from corneal suction cups held in place with mild suction (Figure 3.1). The cup is

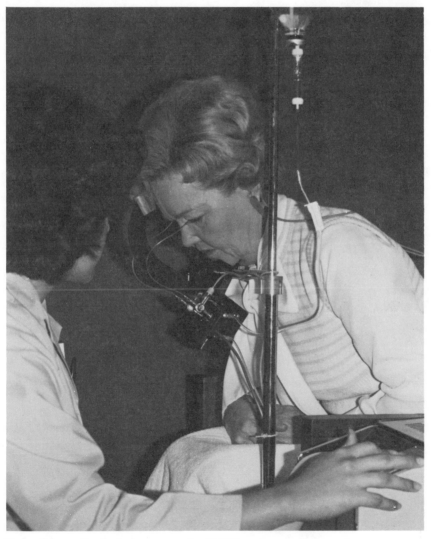

Figure 3.1.   Oculoplethysmography (OPG) test being performed.

gently placed on the anesthetized cornea and mild suction is applied to maintain the cup position. When the cups are in position a closed system is established from the eye to the pressure transducer. The pulse wave is actually a manifestation of the negative pressure exerted when the cornea is withdrawn from the cup as the globe expands with each arterial pulse. Bilateral ocular pulses are recorded simultaneously and the differential between the two pulses is electronically extracted to emphasize the variance between the two eyes. The ocular pulses are recorded together with concomitant external carotid pulses obtained from light opacity earlobe sensors. Delays in timing of these pulses reflect reduction of flow in the internal and/or external carotid artery, respectively.

The test is readily accepted by the patients and is performed without carotid compression or induced ocular hypertension. Systemic hypertension, cardiac arrhythmia, glaucoma, or corneal opacification are not limiting factors for the performance of this test.

Carotid phonoangiography utilizes a specially adapted microphone which is hand held over the cervical carotid arteries (Figure 3.2). The pa-

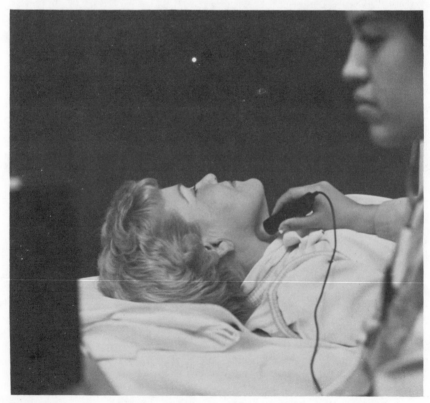

Figure 3.2.   Carotid Phonoangiography (CPA) test being performed.

tient is placed supine to eliminate venous murmurs. Three traces are routinely photographed from each side of the neck: two over the high- and mid-cervical carotid artery to detect bruit of bifurcation origin, and the third at the base of the neck to rule out bruit originating below the carotid bifurcation and radiating up the carotid artery. Multiple exposures are generally used to display the three positional recordings from the same side of the neck on a single photograph. The need is thus eliminated for a physician to auscultate the cervical carotid of each patient since these studies are technician performed with a permanent photographic copy for physician evaluation and analysis.

Interpreting OPG is done by utilizing the differential. The differential is an additional waveform electronically generated by continuously subtracting the amplitude of the left ocular pulse from the right to obtain an algebraic difference. The pulsatility and skewing of this waveform in relation to the ocular pulses emphasizes small differences between the recorded ocular pulses which are not apparent to visual examination. Since the differential waveform is also sensitive to amplitude differences in the ocular pulses, pulsatility of the differential waveform alone does not indicate carotid stenosis (Figure 3.3a). It is the ocular pulse delay as indicated by the shifted or skewed differential waveform relative to the ocular pulse which indicates carotid occlusive disease (Figure 3.3b).

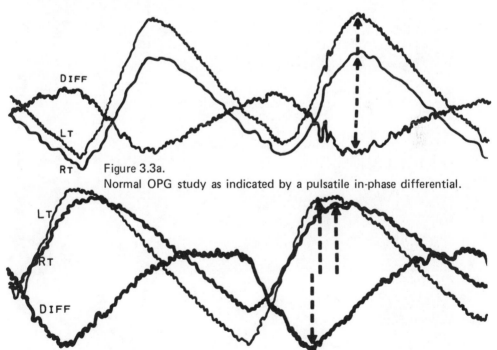

Figure 3.3a.
Normal OPG study as indicated by a pulsatile in-phase differential.

Figure 3.3b. Abnormal OPG study as indicated by a pulsatile out-of-phase differential.

Interpretation of the CPA is based on the extent of blood turbulence which shows as high frequency filling between the first and second heart sounds on the photograph. The significance of the bruit is also determined by its location along the neck. A bruit in the high- and mid-position (Figure 3.4a) is more significant than a bruit at the base of the neck or in the low position (Figure 3.4b).

CLINICAL APPLICATION

The actual OPG/CPA testing generally takes less than 10 min per patient in our laboratory. Much more time is required for scheduling, admitting, taking a limited clinical history, and reporting test results. All testing is done by a nurse or technician with a physician responsible for the final interpretation of the test results. No serious complications or absolute contra-indications have been encountered in the utilization of these tests. During my four-year experience in the laboratory, there have been two mild corneal abrasians which healed spontaneously and two conjunctival hemorrhages

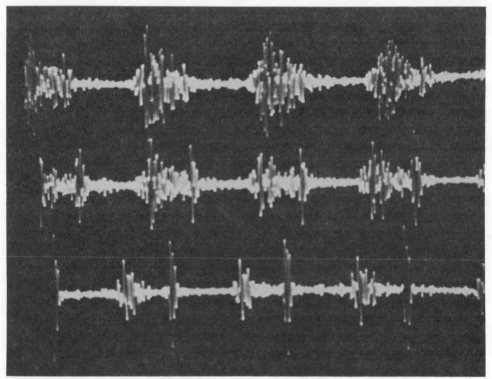

Figure 3.4a.   CPA study indicating significant carotid bifurcational stenosis.

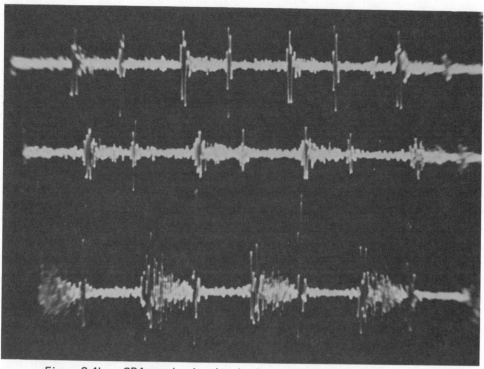

Figure 3.4b. CPA study showing bruit at the base of the neck not indicative of carotid bifurcational stenosis.

relating to this procedure. Testing generally is deferred on patients with obvious eye infection or recent eye surgery until cleared by the referring physician or ophthalmologist.

Ninety percent accuracy has been achieved in our laboratory in detecting significant carotid occlusive disease as documented by greater than 40% stenosis by arteriography.[13]. This is currently based on carotid arteriograms in over one thousand patients. This approximate level of accuracy is also being achieved and reported by other centers.[11,15]

According to Jesse Thompson,[18] 75% of all strokes are caused either by an occlusive or ulcerated lesion in the extracranial vasculature. Only about 40% of the strokes are caused by occlusive lesions and thus these studies may not be sensitive to the remaining 60% unless the emboli producing plaque is stenotic.

Because OPG utilizes the entire carotid system from the aortic arch through the ophthalmic artery, stenoses higher in the internal carotid system above the carotid bifurcation or in the ophthalmic artery are also picked up by this study. These may be considered the largest percentage of false positives, for there is no distinguishing factor to differentiate between these and carotid bifurcational lesions. OPG is not sensitive to ulcerated plaques which throw off small emboli unless these are associated with flow reducing stenoses. However, bruit from nonocclusive ulcerative plaques may be detected by CPA providing a warning for closer patient observation for possible TIA's.

The study has many applications in the field of cerebral vascular disease. It can be used for evaluating patients with TIA's, for screening high-risk patients, for ascertaining origin of carotid bruit, for evaluating progression of carotid disease, for establishing surgical priorities, and for following up patients after carotid endarterectomy. These case studies exemplify many of these applications.

CASE STUDY NO. 1

A 66-year-old lady was initally evaluated as an asymptomatic patient as part of a mass screening study of our hospital personnel and volunteer workers. Initial OPG/CPA studies proved to be negative. The patient was demonstrated to be at risk for a stroke by virtue of recurrent peripheral vascular occlusive disease. Two years later, upon admission for peripheral vascular reconstruction, an asymptomatic carotid bruit was noted and preangiographic OPG/CPA was performed indicating right internal carotid stenosis. The scheduled peripheral vascular reconstruction was deferred because of surgical priority of the carotid stenosis. Carotid arteriography confirmed the presence of a 90% stenosis of the right internal carotid artery. Following uneventful carotid endarterectomy the postoperative evaluation confirmed the restoration of internal carotid artery flow to normal. Subsequently, peripheral vascular reconstruction was performed without incident.

CASE STUDY NO. 2

A similar case is that of a 65-year-old female who volunteered in the early stages of establishing these noninvasive studies. She was negative by the combined studies, with her primary problem being hypertension and a family history of heart disease. She did not have the study repeated annually but returned to the lab three years later by physician referral. At this time she was having TIA's consisting of a numb left arm, occasional dizziness, and pain in her right eye. She remained hypertensive. The OPG/CPA study was very positive, indicating total or near total occlusion of the right internal carotid artery. Arteriography confirmed a total occulsion of the right internal carotid artery with stenosis on the left also. Since a totally occluded artery is not considered operable, the surgeon proceeded with a left carotid endarterectomy. The postoperative study revealed total occlusion on the right as expected and a repeated study at six months revealed no progression of the left internal carotid artery. Today, one and one-half years after surgery, she remains a very active and productive volunteer at a local hospital.

SUMMARY

These noninvasive tests provide an effective, safe, reliable, and inexpensive method for detecting and evaluating extracranial carotid occlusive disease. Advancement in recent years of noninvasive procedures shows great promise in eliminating needless arteriography while preventing disabling strokes.

REFERENCES

1. Barnes RH, Martin GE, Montgomery PS: Ophthalmic plethysmography: techniques and potentials. Dis Nerv Sys, 28:293-297, 1977.

2. Barrios RR, Solis C: Carotid-compression tonographic test — a new method to study the carotid circulation. Acta Neurol Latinoamer, 9:48-67, 1963.

3. Browder A, Browder J: Prevention of stroke. Postgrad Med, 57: 91-97, 1975.

4. Caplan L, Aldredge HR: Diagnosis in cerebrovascular disease. Hosp Med, Feb 1973, pp 84-110.

5. Easton JD, Sherman DG: Stroke and mortality rate in carotid endartectomy: 228 consecutive operations. Stroke, 8:565-568, 1977.

6. Fields WS, Maslenikov V, et al: Joint study of extracranial arterial occlusion. JAMA, 211:1993-2003, 1970.

7. Galin M, Baras I, Cavero R: Ophthalmodynamometry using suction. Arch Ophthal, 81:494-500, 1969.

8. Gee W, Smith CE, et al: Ocular pneumoplethysmography in carotid artery disease. Med Instr, 8:244-8, 1974.

9. Gilroy J, Meyer JS: Auscultation of the neck in occlusive cerebrovascular disease. Circulation, 25:300-310, 1962.

10. Gross M, Popham M: Thermography in vascular disorders affecting the brain. J Neurol Neurosurg Psychiat, 32:484-489, 1969.

11. Gross WS, Verta MJ, et al: Comparison of noninvasive techniques in carotid artery occlusive disease. Surgery, 82:271-279, 1977.

12.   Kartchner MM, McRae LP, Morrison FD: Noninvasive detection and evaluation of carotid occlusive disease. Arch Surg, 106:528-535, 1973.

13.   Kartcher MM, McRae LP, et al: Oculoplethysmography: an adjunct to arteriography in the diagnosis of extracranial carotid occlusive disease. Amer J Surg, 132:728-732, 1976.

14.   Machleder HI, Barker WF: Stroke on the wrong side. Arch Surg, 105:943-947, 1972.

15.   Persson AV: New methods for clinical evaluation of carotid artery disease. Lahey Clin Found Bull, 26:40-43, 1977.

16.   Price TR, Heck AF: Correlation of thermometry and angiography in carotid arterial disease. Arch Neurol, 26:450-455, 1972.

17.   Thomas MH, Petrohelos MS: Diagnostic significance of retinal artery pressure in internal carotid involvement. Amer J Ophthal, 36:335-346, 1953.

18.   Thompson JE, Talkington CM: Carotid endarterectomy. Ann Surg, 184:1-15, 1976.

Challenges in Interpretation of Noninvasive Tests of Cerebrovascular Disease

Robert W. Barnes, MD

Indentification of the stroke-prone patient assumes great importance inasmuch as stroke is the third leading cause of death in this country. More than one-half of all patients who suffer stroke have extracranial arterial occlusive disease as the pathogenic factor. One of the goals in diagnosis of such patients is to identify significant extracranial carotid occlusive disease. The physician may be required to screen patients who have suffered transient ischemic attacks or stroke. In addition many patients harbor significant carotid lesions and are asymptomatic. The traditional method of evaluating such patients is by contrast arteriography which carries a small but potential risk of serious complication, including stroke.

Within the past decade a variety of noninvasive techniques have been developed to detect significant extracranial carotid occlusive disease. One of the major problems of such noninvasive testing is the fact that most techniques are sensitive only to advanced arterial occlusive disease. It is well recognized that the majority of strokes due to extracranial occlusive disease occur on the basis of emboli from the arterial plaques. Such emboli may emanate from ulceration or thrombosis on nonobstructing lesions. It is thus incumbent on the physician to recognize the limitation of noninvasive testing and to integrate such modalities with care into the management of stroke-prone patients.

TECHNIQUES

Although many noninvasive tests have been developed for detection of extracranial carotid occlusive disease, there are three techniques that are most commonly used: 1) Doppler ultrasound, 2) plethysmography, and 3) phono-angiography.

DOPPLER ULTRASOUND

Instrumentation. Many Doppler instruments are available, but most techniques for cerebrovascular screening involve continuous-wave instruments. A directionally-sensitive Doppler detector is particularly useful for detection of cerebrovascular disease. The instrument permits determination of directional blood flow using the output of stereo-earphones, the deflection of a panel meter needle, the deflection of recording above or below a zero baseline, or the presence or absence of flow depending upon the depression of a probe selection switch. In addition to continuous wave instruments, pulsed-Doppler ultrasound has proved useful to image the carotid bifurcation noninvasively. Such pulse-Doppler instruments are sensitive to the depth or range of detected blood flow distal to the transducer.

Methods. There are three basic techniques of using Doppler ultrasound to detect extracranial carotid occlusive disease:

1.   Periorbital Doppler examination

2.   Carotid Doppler examination

3.   Noninvasive Doppler ultrasonic arteriography

Periorbital Doppler examination involves assessment of directional blood flow in the peripheral branches of each ophthalmic artery (frontal, supra-orbital and nasal arteries). Normally blood flow is directed out of the eye and is augmented by compression of various branches of the external carotid artery (superficial temporal, infraorbital and facial arteries). In the presence of significant extracranial carotid occlusive disease, the ophthalmic artery may carry reversed flow via the extracranial branches of the external carotid artery. Detection of such extracranial collateral flow is possible by noting attenuation of periorbital reversed arterial flow signals in response to compression of one of the branches of the external carotid arteries. In addition, intracranial collateral circulation from the opposite internal carotid artery may be determined by transient common carotid artery compression low in the neck (to avoid stimulating carotid baroreceptors or dislodgement of emboli from a diseased carotid bifurcation). To distinguish stenosis (operable) from occlusion (inoperable) of the internal carotid artery, a direct examination of the flow signals from the common, external and internal carotid arteries in the neck may be performed by audible, analogue tracing or sound spectral analysis. Noninvasive carotid imaging is possible by translating detected flow velocity information, using a continuous or pulse Doppler, to a storage oscilloscope by means of a position-sensing arm. Such noninvasive images permit determination of areas of stenosis or occlusions of branches of the carotid artery. In addition, the Doppler imaging detector also permits recording of flow velocity signals for subsequent analogue tracings or sound spectral analysis.

Plethysmography. A variety of plethysmographic techniques have been developed to detect significant extracranial carotid occlusive disease. Most devices have involved application of a water or air-filled transducer to the

74

anesthetized eye. The water-filled ocular plethysmograph (OPG) permits recording of ocular pulse waveforms. Delay in the ocular pulse tracing is an indication of significant extracranial carotid occlusive disease. An air-filled oculopneumoplethysmograph permits determination of ocular blood pressure for detection of extracranial carotid occlusive disease as well as hemispheric collateral blood pressure.

The photoplethysmograph is a new technique to determine supra-orbital pulsation in response to compression of extracranial branches of each external carotid artery as well as each common carotid artery. This technique is rapid and sensitive to significant extracranial carotid occlusive disease. Although a number of false-positive examinations may occur, the technique is useful to screen large numbers of patients for carotid disease. An attribute of the technique is the fact that the transducers are not applied to the eye.

Phonoangiography. Although the carotid bruit is a frequent sign of significant extracranial carotid occlusive disease, previously no method was available to objectively record the intensity and duration of the bruit. The phonoangiograph permits a graphic representation of the amplitude and duration of the bruit by means of recording the tracing of a storage oscilloscope on a Polaroid photograph. The technique is useful to discriminate carotid from radiating bruits, to define hemodynamically significant internal carotid stenoses (bruit extending into diastole) and to detect minor lesions not identified by a conventional stethoscope.

APPLICATIONS AND INTERPRETATIONS

Noninvasive evaluation of cerebrovascular disease is applicable to several types of patients. The most useful categories of individuals helped by non-invasive cerebrovascular screening are: 1) symptomatic patients with cerebral ischemia; 2) patients with asymptomatic disease; 3) patients at high-risk in screening studies; 4) monitoring of patients during operation; 5) postoperative monitoring of patients; 6) determination of hemispheric collateral blood pressure.

Symptomatic Disease. Patients with symptoms of hemispheric or vertebrobasilar transient ischemic attacks or stroke are candidates for contrast arteriography. Although noninvasive techniques are useful to identify significant extracranial occlusive disease of the internal carotid artery, many patients with symptoms of cerebral ischemia have normal noninvasive screening evaluations. Such patients may have nonobstructing extracranial carotid lesions which are a source of emboli, but are not of sufficient severity to present a hemodynamic obstruction to the carotid circulation. Some patients have nonlateralizing symptoms such as dizziness, syncope or memory disturbance. Such patients may be screened for significant carotid occlusive disease by noninvasive techniques. Patients who have a normal examination are unlikely to have lesions which can be operatively corrected to the benefit of the patient. Conversely some patients with nonlateralizing, ambiguous cerebrovascular symptoms have extensive carotid lesions which, when corrected, may render the patient asymptomatic or considerably improved.

Asymptomatic Disease. Many patients with significant carotid occlusive disease are asymptomatic. Often such patients have a carotid bruit detectable by the standard stethoscope. However some patients have bruits which can only be identified by phonoangiography. Another group of patients has significant extracranial carotid occlusive disease in the absence of a bruit (particularly patients with internal carotid occlusion). Such patients can be screened by noninvasive techniques and the lesions identified. Such detection of asymptomatic disease may assume importance in patients who undergo major operative procedures for correction of an unrelated condition (resection of an abdominal aortic aneurysm, coronary bypass grafting).

Screening of High-Risk Patients. Patients who have carotid occlusive disease may fall into several types of high-risk groups. Such patients include those with coronary artery occlusive disease, patients with hyperlipidemia, diabetic patients, hypertensive individuals and patients with a strong family history of stroke or cardiovascular disease. Such patients may be screened at periodic intervals for carotid lesions, although the therapeutic implications of detected disease remains controversial.

Monitoring of Therapy. Patients who undergo operation for carotid occlusive disease are monitored in a variety of ways. The most standard technique is intraoperative monitoring of the electroencephalogram. However other techniques are available, including measurement of carotid artery back (stump) pressure. A useful technique is the assessment of carotid artery flow velocity signals using a sterile Doppler probe. In addition, supraorbital photoplethysmography is possible throughout a carotid operation. Finally, a periorbital Doppler exam is a useful technique to ascertain the integrity of a carotid endarterectomy prior to closure of the operative wound.

Postoperative Evaluation. Patients who undergo carotid endarterectomy may be screened by noninvasive techniques in the immediate postoperative period. Most patients should have a normal cerebrovascular examination following carotid endarterectomy. An occasional patient (less than 5%) may suffer an asymptomatic occlusion of the internal carotid artery, which may be detected noninvasively. The decision to reoperate on such patients remains controversial. Patients who develop a stroke during or immediately following operation should be rapidly screened by noninvasive techniques. If a carotid occlusion is detected by a noninvasive examination, consideration may be given to immediate reoperation without awaiting the performance of arteriography with a resultant time delay. Postoperative serial noninvasive studies are useful to determine the continued integrity of carotid reconstructions and to detect disease progression or postoperative complications.

Hemispheric Collateral Blood Pressure. Measurement of collateral hemispheric blood pressure is a useful index of the adequacy of collateral pathways to a hemisphere involved by temporary or permanent occlusion of the carotid artery. Such decisions are useful in the planning of major procedures on the head and neck. In addition the technique is useful to predict whether or not a patient will suffer a catastrophic insult following occlusion of an internal carotid artery. Although hemispheric collateral blood pressure may be determined by oculopneumoplethysmography, the adequacy of such pressure may be estimated by Doppler ultrasound. In patients who continue to have normal directional flow in the ophthalmic artery during transient common carotid artery compression, the carotid back (stump) pressure is always greater than 50 mm Hg. Patients who have obliteration of the ophthalmic artery flow or reversion to reverse flow during common carotid compression nearly always have a low carotid back pressure (<50 mm/Hg) at the time of operation.

CONCLUSIONS

Although contrast arteriography remains the diagnostic standard for symptomatic patients with transient ischemic attacks or stroke, many patients are candidates for noninvasive screening of the cerebrovascular circulation. Such patients include those who have asymptomatic carotid bruits, patients with predisposing factors to stroke, patients who undergo carotid endarterectomy and patients with nonspecific cerebrovascular dysfunction such as dizziness, syncope or memory disturbance. Such patients may be screened by Doppler examination or ocular plethysmography and further studies may be applicable if such tests are abnormal. The physician must recognize that many episodes of cerebral ischemia result from nonobstructing plaques which are not detectable by conventional noninvasive screening techniques. Such patients deserve contrast arteriography to identify operable lesions. However noninvasive techniques are useful to screen asymptomatic or ambiguous patients for significant carotid occlusive disease. Although conventional noninvasive techniques may not distinguish operable stenoses from inoperable occlusions, the development of ultrasonic arteriography has permitted increased accuracy of the definition of clinically significant carotid occlusions in the stroke-prone patient.

Section 4

Patient Conditioning

This area of patient care is indeed coming into its own as a recognized adjunct to the medical and surgical care of a patient with heart disease. Cardiac conditioning programs are being initiated throughout the country, and not without due justification. Exercise has been shown by many investigators to enhance physical performance and improve the quality of life in heart-diseased patients, though its direct effect upon the incidence and progression of atherosclerotic heart disease has not been determined.

For the postsurgical patient, it is imperative that he regain and even improve his physical stamina as soon after surgery as possible. A quick return to physical activity is encouraging to the patient, augmenting his compliance to postsurgical therapies and improving his mental and emotional outlook.

In the immediate postoperative period, pulmonary conditioning is vital to the health of the lungs. As the patient progresses, conditioning may begin slowly with walking and moderately exertional exercises, a program similar to that of the postmyocardial infarction patient. Cardiac conditioning may begin as soon as the patient is physically able to be safely tested for his maximum exercise tolerance. From this information, the exercise physiologist can prescribe an exercise program to guide the patient safely and confidently through a gradual enhancement of his performance capabilities. In most instances, the patient experiences a psychological improvement also from the realization that he is in control of his improving health.

In this section there are several papers which offer an excellent overview of the various aspects of patient conditioning. Pulmonary conditioning for both the postoperative patient and the person afflicted with lung disease is presented in an educational paper delineating the procedures available to the respiratory therapist. The next paper deals with the special considerations a postmyocardial infarction patient must be given as regards a return to daily activities. This paper also offers a review of current literature on the subject.

The latter two papers are highly informative reviews of exercise physiology fundamentals and the use of these principles in the composition of an exercise prescription for the postsurgical patient. Instruction is offered in how an exercise program is structured for the individual, as well as the general procedures used in cardiac conditioning protocols.

Chronic Responses to Exercise

Jack H. Wilmore, PhD

Physiological responses to exercise may be categorized into acute and chronic adaptations. Acute responses are those which occur with a single episode of work, while chronic adaptations result from a period of physical conditioning. It is the latter type of response which I wish to discuss, but limited to the cardiovascular and metabolic aspects.

Assuming a previously sedentary person begins a 3-day-a-week, 20-minute-per-day jogging program, working at 75% of his endurance capacity, his resting heart rate will be reduced by approximately one beat/min for each of the initial 10 to 15 weeks he is active in the program. Resting heart rates of 40 beats/min are not uncommon in highly trained athletes. Training produces little change in the maximal heart rate, although Pollock[1] suggests that there is a tendency for maximal heart rate to decrease with training if the maximal heart rate was initally above 180 beats/min. Nevertheless, maximal heart rate is more closely associated with age than physical condition.[2] During standardized, submaximal bouts of exercise, the heart rate will be considerably lower following a training period. Likewise, postexercise recovery rates will be significantly lower following either standardized submaximal or maximal exercise periods.

Associated with the changes in resting, exercise, and recovery heart rates are the inversely proportional changes of similar magnitude in stroke volume. The stroke volume at rest, during standardized, submaximal exercise and at maximal exercise is increased as a result of training. However, the combined effects of stroke volume and heart rate include little or no change in the cardiac output ($\dot{Q}$) at rest or during submaximal exercise, but produce a considerable increase in maximum cardiac output ($\dot{Q}_{max}$). Pretraining $\dot{Q}_{max}$ values of 18 to 20 liters/min may be increased to 23 to 25 liters/min following conditioning. Values as high as 42 liters/min have been reported in highly trained, endurance athletes.[3]

Heart volume and weight also undergo a slight increase during training. Once considered a pathologic condition, cardiac hypertrophy, "athlete's heart," is now proclaimed a normal response to the continual stress of exercise.[4] Blood volume is also augmented, as is total hemoglobin, although the hematocrit will remain unchanged or be slightly reduced due to increased plasma volume.

Training of the normal individual probably has little influence on resting arterial blood pressure, but it may cause a decrease in pressure in the hypertensive subject.[1] Peripheral blood flow is affected by training due to an apparently greater density of capillaries in the active muscles,[3] thus providing better perfusion in the muscle and greater total blood supply during maximal levels of exercise.

Pulmonary ventilation is lowered at standardized, submaximal exercise but greatly increased during maximal levels of work following training.[1] Pulmonary diffusion is affected only at maximal exercise. The resulting increase is thought attributable to enhanced lung perfusion from greater pulmonary blood flow in the upper regions of the lung.[5]

Oxygen consumption ($\dot{V}O_2$) at rest and at standardized, submaximal levels of exercise is either unaltered or marginally reduced following conditioning. Maximum oxygen consumption ($\dot{V}O_{2max}$) is substantially increased following endurance training, however. Rises of from 4% to 93% have been reported, but most authors indicate a range of from 15% to 30%.[1]

The factors responsible for this increase in $\dot{V}O_2$ max have been identified, but there is considerable controversy over their relative importance. Logical arguments have been raised to support the concept that a substantial portion of the change in $\dot{V}O_{2\,max}$ is the result of alterations in size, number, and content of the muscle mitochondria, i.e., $\dot{V}O_{2\,max}$ is limited by the oxidative capacity of the muscle cell and not by the inadequate supply of oxygen to the mitochondria.[6] Others[7,8,9] support the more traditional view that $\dot{V}O_{2\,max}$ is restricted by $\dot{Q}_{max}$ and local tissue perfusion, i.e., there is an inadequate supply of oxygen being delivered to the active tissue. A recent review on the efficacy of oxygen as a work facilitating agent demonstrated that oxygen breathing increased maximal work performance by approximately the same percentage as the increase in the partial pressure of oxygen.[10]

There is apparently a limit as to what levels $\dot{V}O_{2\,max}$ can attain with training, and this is undoubtedly influenced by heredity.[3] However, it does appear that one's performance can continue to improve through the development of a sustained work pace which reflects a higher percentage of $\dot{V}O_{2\,max}$.

As a result of endurance training, important physiological changes take place which facilitate the delivery of oxygen to the active muscles during submaximal and maximal exercise. Table 4.1 lists typical values before and after a training program for a number of physiological and body composition parameters. For comparative purposes, the values for a world class endurance runner are shown. These figures illustrate the tremendous adaptability of man, as well as the great difference in values between a trained normal individual and a highly trained, skilled athlete. The latter phenomenon is due to basic genetic differences between individuals, demonstrating that endurance athletic performance is an innate capacity. Training can take one only to his or her potential genetic limit.

TABLE 4.1
Hypothetical Physiological and Body Composition Changes in a Sedentary Normal Individual Resulting from an Endurance Training Program,* Compared to the Values of a World Class Endurance Runner of the Same Age

Variables	Sedentary Normal Pretraining	Sedentary Normal Post-training	World Class Endurance Runner
Cardiovascular			
HR_{rest}, beats/min	71	59	36
HR_{max}, beats/min	185	183	174
SV_{rest}, ml†	65	80	125
SV_{max}, ml†	120	140	200
$\dot{Q}_{rest}$, liters/min	4.6	4.7	4.5
$\dot{Q}_{max}$, liters/min	22.2	25.6	34.8
Heart volume, ml	750	820	1,200
Blood volume, liters	4.7	5.1	6.0
Systolic BP_{rest}, mmHg	135	130	120
Systolic BP_{max}, mmHg	210	205	210
Diastolic BP_{rest}, mmHg	78	76	65
Diastolic BP_{max}, mmHg	82	80	65
Respiratory			
$\dot{V}_{E\,rest}$, liters/min (BTPS)	7	6	6
$\dot{V}_{E\,max}$, liters/min (BTPS)	110	135	195
f_{rest}, breaths/min	14	12	12
f_{max}, breaths/min	40	45	55
TV_{rest}, liters	0.5	0.5	0.5
TV_{max}, liters			3.5
VC, liters	5.8	6.0	6.2
RV, liters	1.4	1.2	1.2
Metabolic			
a $\overline{V}O_2$ diff$_{rest}$, ml/100 ml	6.0	6.0	6.0
a $\overline{V}O_2$ diff$_{max}$, ml/100 ml			16.0
$\dot{V}O_{2\,rest}$, ml/kg · min	3.5	3.7	4.0
$\dot{V}O_{2\,max}$, ml/kg · min	40.5	49.8	76.7
Blood lactate$_{rest}$, mg/100 ml	10	10	10
Blood lactate$_{max}$, mg/100 ml	110	125	185
Body Composition			
Weight, lbs	175	170	150
Fat weight, lbs	28	21.3	11.3
Lean weight, lbs	147	148.7	138.7
Relative fat, %	16.0	12.5	7.5

* 6-month training program, jogging 3 to 4 times/week, 30 min/day, at 75% of his $\dot{V}O_2$ max

† Upright position

Reproduced with permission from Wilmore JH, Norton AC: The Heart and Lungs at Work: A Primer of Exercise Physiology, Schiller Park, Illinois: Beckman Instruments, 1974.

REFERENCES

1. Pollock ML: The quantification of endurance training programs, in Wilmore, JH Ed, Exercise and Sport Sciences Reviews, Vol 1, New York, Academic Press, 1973, pp 155-88.

2. Fox SM, Haskell WL: The exercise stress test: needs for standardization in Cardiology: Current Topics and Progress, New York, Academic Press, 1970, p 149.

3. Åstrand P-O, Rodahl K: Textbook of Work Physiology, 2nd ed, New York, McGraw-Hill, 1977.

4. Barnard RJ: Long-term effects of exercise on cardiac function, in Wilmore, JH Ed, Exercise and Sport Sciences Reviews, Vol 3, New York, Academic Press, 1975, pp 113-33.

5. Wilmore JH, Norton AC: The Heart and Lungs at Work: A Primer of Exercise Physiology, Schiller Park, Illinois, Beckman Instruments, 1974.

6. Holloszy JO: Biochemical adaptations to exercise: aerobic metabolism, in Wilmore, JH Ed, Exercise and Sport Sciences Reviews, Vol. 1, New York, Academic Press, 1973, pp 45-71.

7. Prinay F, Dujardin J, Derdanne R, et al: Muscular exercise during intoxication by carbon monoxide. J Appl Physiol, 31:373-5, 1871.

8. Ekblom BJ, Goldbarg AN, Gullbring B: Response to exercise after blood loss and reinfusion. J Appl Physiol, 33: 175-80, 1972.

9. Kaijser J: On the limiting factors for heavy exercise in normal man, in Larsen, OA and Malmborg, RO Eds, Coronary Heart Disease and Physical Fitness, Baltimore, University Park Press, 1971, p 41.

10. Wilmore JH: Oxygen, in Morgan, WP Ed, Ergogenic Aids and Muscular Performance, New York, Academic Press, 1972, pp 321-43.

Abstracted with permission from Amsterdam EA, Wilmore JH, and DeMaria AN Eds, Exercise in Cardiovascular Health and Diseases, New York, Yorke Medical Books, 1977. Copyright © 1977 by Yorke Medical Books, a division of Dun-Donnelley Publishing Corporation.

Concepts of Pulmonary Rehabilitation

Caroline M. Hughes, RN

Rehabilitation or long term therapy of the pulmonary patient has been accomplished in the past through various types of breathing apparati and therapy modes. Today, technology has advanced so that we may individualize an oxygen treatment program to the total needs of the patient. Rehabilitation of the pulmonary patient involves a total body concept, one that strives to provide adequate oxygen supplementation during periods of both rest and exertion. The goal is to help recondition the patient's body for optimal oxygen utilization through a six-phase therapy approach: activity-related oxygen supplementation, graded exercise, alternative breathing patterns, medication, heart rate/body weight monitoring, and postural drainage.

THEORY AND METHODOLOGY

In the normal lung, oxygenation of the blood occurs through the exchange of oxygen for carbon dioxide within the capillaries bordering the alveolar sacs. If the lung becomes diseased so that oxygen does not reach the alveolar sacs in sufficient quantity, the level of carbon dioxide in the blood increases along with the number of red blood cells. This then changes the pH of the blood, making it more acidic, and may cause a shift in the metabolic pathway. The object then, in treating the pulmonary patient, is to deliver enough oxygen to the lungs to maintain an adequate oxygen saturation level in the blood, thereby eliminating the metabolic aberrations induced by oxygen deprivation.

To measure the oxygen saturation levels in pulmonary patients we use the ear oximeter. This computerized, colorimetric device allows oxygen determinations even while the patient exercises, a considerable improvement over earlier, more cumbersome procedures. A light source and fiberoptic probe are placed on either side of the pinna of the ear, since arterial and venous oxygen saturation levels are nearly equal at this point. Data supplied by the probe is analyzed by the computer and oxygen saturation levels are determined. Readings are taken at rest and while the patient exercises on a bicycle ergometer or treadmill. If desaturation occurs, oxygen is administered at measured flow rates until adequate saturation is achieved. Thus, an oxygen prescription is obtained from this information, and the patient can now achieve a prescribed activity level while maintaining adequate oxygenation.

Once the oxygen requirements are defined, the patient may adjust his or her supply according to the exertional levels of various activities. This helps prevent misuse or abuse of the oxygen supply. To further assist the patient in attaining adequate oxygen saturation, we teach lateral costal breathing techniques. Moreover, we instruct the patient on the names and use of his or her medications and the monitoring techniques for his or her heart rate and body weight. Last among our six-phase program is the extremely important aspect of pulmonary drainage. Maintaining adequate pulmonary toilet is vital; accumulated secretions in the trachobronchial tree interfere with oxygenation. We teach the patient four basic positions, but others may be used. We suggest a booklet (*Better Living and Breathing. A Manual for Patients*, Modrak and Moser, C. V. Mosby Co., St. Louis, 1975) which is an excellent guide to pulmonary drainage. One must be aware of other non-pulmonary conditions which may pose a problem with certain body positions, so one must keep in mind the total medical aspect when explaining postural drainage techniques.

DISCUSSION

Successful rehabilitation of the pulmonary patient involves a great deal of patient education and team work among physicians, nurses, and respiratory therapists. With today's equipment and prescription techniques, the patient can improve his or her physical condition and hopefully enhance his or her quality of life.

The cardiopulmonary department of our hospital offers a service to the pulmonary patient that is unique in its concept. This six-phase rehabilitation program has shown excellent results in the past few years, and many private physicians have availed themselves of our services in the treatment of their pulmonary patients.

Patient Education:
Postmyocardial Infarction
A Review of the Literature

Susan Sherbocker, RN, CVS

In recent years there has been much concern in the health field regarding patient education. That patients not only have a desire for, but a right to, health education is illustrated in "A Patient's Bill of Rights." Drafted by the American Hospital Association in 1973, it states that:

The patient has the right to obtain from his physician complete current information concerning his diagnosis, treatment and prognosis in terms the patient can be reasonably expected to understand.

Involving the hospital, the Bill continues with:

The patient has the right to expect that the hospital will provide a mechanism whereby he is informed by his physician or a delegate of the physician of the patient's continuing health care requirements following discharge.

This brings us, as nurses, or delegates of the physician, into the realm of discharge planning and teaching. The patient who has survived a myocardial infarction is one with many specific educational needs prior to and after discharge from the hospital.

Therefore, certain questions must be answered if the hospital is to provide this mechanism for the discharge planning and continued education of the MI patient.

The first question is, "WHAT IS PATIENT EDUCATION?"

According to Ulrich, "Patient education should consist of organized health education experiences, planned by physicians, professional health workers, and the patient himself to meet the patient's specific learning needs, interests, and capabilities, and offered as an integral part of the patient's total health care."

This definition incorporates many components essential to a successful educational program. First of all, it stresses that an organized approach must be used. The educational program must be planned, rather than left to chance. Otherwise there is the chance that nothing will be done.

The patient himself is to be involved as an active participant in the teaching-learning process. His specific learning needs, not the teacher's, must be identified and the program must be individualized to take into account his interests and his capabilities.

One example of a cardiac teaching program which meets these criteria can be found at Grady Memorial Hospital in Atlanta, Ga. Here the health teachers are dealing with an indigent population and their program is adapted to deal with the specific needs of these patients. The printed material used is written so that the patient is able to read and understand it. The dietary instructions given take into consideration the foods that the patient likes and is able to buy — for example, salt pork.

Finally, Ulrich's definition identifies education as an "integral part" of total patient care. Thus, it is listed as a priority in the nursing care plan. No longer should we assign giving a bath or making a bed a greater priority than teaching our patient to be able to assume responsibility for his or her health care.

"WHY IS IT IMPORTANT TO EDUCATE THE PATIENT WHO HAD SUSTAINED A MYOCARDIAL INFARCTION?"

The answers to this question seem obvious and are closely related to the goals of the educational program. They are well-defined in the literature.[14, 16, 17, 26, 29] While the patient is in-hospital:

1. Education is felt to decrease the patient's and family's anxieties. Increased knowledge and understanding helps both to overcome their fears of the unknown regarding, initially, what has happened and, later on, how this will affect their life styles.

2. Education increases cooperation in the Coronary Care Unit. The patient who understands that his activities are restricted at this time to promote healing of his heart is more likely to comply with these restrictions. And, the nurse should realize that a cooperative patient increases the likelihood that medical intervention may be able to limit the infarct size and prevent complications.

3. Royle and Cassem feel that education promotes the psychological adaptation of the MI patient thus preventing chronic depression and cardiac invalidism. They feel that rehabilitation programs, incorporating progressive, supervised physical activity and education, should begin no later than the third CCU day. This is the time at which most MI patients experience the onset of depression.

Studies have shown that most patients retain only one-fourth to one-third of the information presented to them while in the hospital.[22] Therefore, it is important to continue the educational program on an outpatient basis. For patients enrolled in a cardiac conditioning (exercise) program, an ideal setting is provided for continued patient and family education.

Regarding discharge instruction and teaching programs presented on an outpatient basis after the patient has left the hospital environment:

1. Education helps to increase patient compliance with prescribed medical therapy. It is not enough for the physician or the health educator to merely tell the patient that he must stop smoking, change his dietary habits, control stressful situations, and take his medications as prescribed. We must remember that the patient is an adult, not a child. He needs to understand the importance of making these changes. This approach allows the patient to feel respected and to become a part of the health care team.

2. Education helps to dispel the patient's myths and misconceptions about heart disease which he encounters by seeking information from friends and acquaintances with similar problems when health teachers have not made correct information available to him.

3. Through education we hope to prevent complications which could lead to rehospitalization or even death. We need to stress the importance of seeking help should the situation arise in order to prevent costly delays.

4. Lastly, although we cannot guarantee it, through cardiac rehabilitation programs we hope to prevent the recurrence of myocardial infarction and promote the return to as near normal life as possible for the patient. Through education of family members, we hope to decrease the incidence of MI in this high-risk group.

Thus the overall goal of a cardiac teaching program is to promote health through learning. The health of both patient and family is promoted through the teaching of preventive measures. Learning, of course, can only be measured by changes in attitude and changes in behavior.

"WHO SHOULD TEACH THE MI PATIENT?"

Actually, the term physician means "teacher." Historically, any information a patient was given was presented by his physician. With the increased demands made on physicians today, they have little time to fulfill this role as teacher. Therefore, other medical and paramedical personnel have begun to aid the physician in the education of his patient. Today nurses, pharmacists, dieticians and other health practitioners, including one group specially trained in teaching techniques — the health educators — are all actively involved in educational programs.

This team approach seems to work best in cardiac teaching programs. Several factors remain important to the effectiveness of this approach, however.

First the patient's primary care physician must be aware of and in agreement with that which is being taught. The physician needs to inform the patient that he has referred him to the teaching program and that he supports the materials being presented.

Nothing could be worse than to present the patient with information which is contradictory to his physician's instructions. This places the patient in a real dilemma. At best, he could decide that only his physician knows what he is talking about and choose to comply with his advice. At worst, he may decide that no one knows what he is talking about and choose to rely on his own "common sense" regarding continued health care. In either case, the patient has not been helped, and education has not been effective.

Needless to say, the teachers involved in the educational program must have a thorough knowledge of the materials they plan to present. However, a knowledge of teaching techniques and adult learning behaviors is also important. The teaching approach used will greatly affect the outcome: in other words, learning.

Patients have related that the single most important criterion for any teacher is empathy.[13] Without this quality the effectiveness of any teaching program is diminished.

"IS THE PATIENT THE ONLY ONE WHO NEEDS TO BE INVOLVED IN THE CARDIAC TEACHING PROGRAM?"

In one study it was hypothesized that the patients whose spouses had the most knowledge and understanding of heart disease and its treatment would show the best compliance with recommended therapy.[40] This hypothesis proved incorrect, however, and it was shown that the patient himself must be presented with the information and the ultimate responsiblity for his continued health care.

This does not mean that the spouse should be excluded from the cardiac teaching program. The fact that spouses have very specific, although somewhat different, learning needs has also been documented.[2,37]

Spouses, as well as family members, must have a thorough understanding of coronary heart disease in order to provide an atmosphere of support and become a positive influence in the patient's recovery. All must agree, however, that the ultimate responsibility for acceptance or rejection of medical recommendations lies with the patient.

As mentioned previously, offspring, siblings and their families must be included in the learner group. Prevention and the early detection and treatment of heart disease needs to be emphasized.

One group which has been identified but seldom included in cardiac teaching programs is the general public. They must be taught to recognize, and know what to do for, the early warning signs of heart attack. They need an understanding of the detection and modification of coronary risk factors. And, most important to our patient, employers, unions, and insurance agencies need an understanding of the MI victim. They must realize that he can and should return to work as soon as his physician indicates he is able.

"WHAT INFORMATION NEEDS TO BE TAUGHT?"

As discussed previously, any educational program must be individualized to meet the learner's specific needs. However, there is general agreement regarding the content of cardiac teaching programs.[1,4,15,17,22,30,36] These topics can be outlined as follows:

1. General informaton
   a. normal heart function
   b. ischemic heart disease
   c. definition of medical terms

2. Coronary risk factors
   a. control of associated medical conditions, i.e., hypertension and diabetes
   b. cessation of smoking
   c. identification and modification of risk factors for relatives
   d. control of stress

3. Physical activity
   a. relation of early activity restrictions to the healing process
   b. specific instructions about activity while the patient is in the hospital and after discharge, including frank discussions regarding resuming sexual activity and returning to employment
   c. discussion of energy-conserving methods
   d. rationale for a safe physical reconditioning program, including recommended types of exercises as well as those to be avoided (isometrics), the basis for an exercise prescription, and benefits the patient can hope to achieve.

4. Nutrition
   a. reduction of calories and fats to decrease obesity and reduce the work of the heart
   b. principles and practice of sodium restriction if necessary
   c. explanation of methods to reduce serum cholesterol levels (if these are found to be elevated)

5. Medications
    a. name
    b. purpose
    c. dosage
    d. side effects
    e. special instructions regarding skipping doses, taking extra doses, taking with meals or on an empty stomach, precautions about alcohol, etc.
    f. information about special identification tags (Coumadin)
6. Medical care after discharge
    a. identification of patient's own warning system
    b. discussion of emergency procedure to avoid delay in seeking care; CPR for family members
    c. medical vs surgical aspects
7. Psychological aspects
    a. assist patient and family to realize that anger, denial, guilt, and depression are normal coping mechanisms
    b. provide resources for assisting psychological adaptation.

"HOW CAN WE ASSESS OUR PATIENT'S READINESS TO LEARN?"

Research has indicated that it is a mistake to wait until a patient asks questions before beginning a teaching program. It is felt that the lack of requesting specific information may be related to fear, denial, or an inadequate understanding of what the patient thinks he needs to know. Patients have indicated that even though they did not ask any questions, they still expected to be provided with any information that was necessary for them to know before discharge from the hospital.

Several sources refer to the fact that different learning needs must be met during the various stages of psychological adaptation.[1,5,18,23,27,37,44]

The idea has also been presented that, in order for teachers to be effective, the problems the patient identifies are those which must be met. However, what about those problems health educators identify by virtue of their knowledge and experience? According to Bryan: "These must first become a problem in the patient's understanding if the teacher is to have his cooperation and involvement in solving them. In other words, his attitudes, feelings and beliefs must first be changed before he can be motivated towards constructive action."

Therefore, what motivates an adult towards learning, i.e. changing his attitudes, feelings, and beliefs? The adult is motivated by the problems he experiences in life and thinks may be alleviated through education. There is a time perspective of immediacy of application to his problem solving.[24] The person who has just experienced an MI (and is past the denial phase) is usually highly motivated towards learning.

"HOW CAN A CARDIAC TEACHING PROGRAM BE IMPLEMENTED IN THE HOSPITAL SETTING?"

The program must be individualized as much to the institution as to the patient. Anyone wishing to implement a cardiac teaching program must first have a knowledge of the hospital system as well as the support of its administration and physicians.

Research of the literature and contact with hospitals similar to one's own is beneficial regarding programs already established. If possible, it is very helpful to visit other institutions and observe their programs.

The teaching methods which can be used are numerous. Individual and group instruction have been successful and a combination of the two seems to achieve the best results.

Audiovisual aides are usually necessary to enhance the effectiveness of the learning process. One study showed that patients were much more likely to complete a program when it was presented by videotape as opposed to straight lecture.[11]

Audiovisuals can be made by the teachers or purchased from other institutions, free-lance producers, corporations specializing in the production of materials or from the local heart association. Those materials reported as best meeting the needs of various programs include (1) printed materials — pamphlets, booklets and programmed instructional units; (2) audiotapes; (3) videotapes and programs for closed circuit television; (4) slide presentations; (5) flipcharts; and (6) models showing heart structure and the process of atherosclerosis.

Once teaching plans have been written and the teaching methods determined, a means of documentation and evaluation must be established. Some hospitals have developed special forms kept in the patient's chart or on a clipboard at the foot of his bed for recording instructions which have been completed and for recording assessment of the patient's understanding of the material. Others have used the problem-oriented medical record for documentation purposes.

Methods of evaluation which have been suggested include (1) objective pretests and posttests to determine teaching effectiveness; (2) subjective evaluation forms sent to learner participants at specific intervals following completion of the educational program; (3) telephone calls to participants requesting information regarding behavior change and compliance with therapy; and (4) evaluation forms sent to the patient's physician requesting specific information regarding medical compliance.

The next problem which needs to be solved is that of cost and budget. In some settings the patient is charged a fee for this service; in others, it is considered a part of his total care. Skillern feels that patient education will eventually be partly or completely reimbursable through third-party arrangements (the government or private insurance agencies), provided it is presented through an accredited institution.

Now the teaching program is ready to be implemented. It should be given a trial of three to six months and then, based on the evaluations, revisions and changes can be made. The program will continue to need reevaluation and revision at certain intervals to obtain optimal results.

Finally, what has been the physician and patient response to these educational programs? In general, the responses of physicians have ranged from enthusiastic to resistant. Patients and their families have been overwhelmingly receptive and appreciative for these learning opportunities.

What, then, about the nurse or health educator? Bryan's comments seem most appropriate: "Teaching patients and families is not easy. It is complex and challenging and involves the investment of time and emotional energy, but helping people recognize their health needs and understand ways of meeting them is an essential responsibility of every nurse in whatever setting she works."

The only question which remains to be answered is:

"WHAT ARE YOU DOING ABOUT PATIENT EDUCATION?"

BIBLIOGRAPHY

1. Abram H. Emotional responses to heart disease. Cardiac Pacemaker, Inc., 21-22, October, 1977. Short article outlining emotional responses of the postsurgical cardiac and post-MI patient.

2. Adsett CA, Gruhn, JG. Short-term group psychotherapy for post-myocardial infarction patients and their wives. The Canadian Medical Association Journal, 99:577-584, Sept. 28, 1968. A study of six cardiac patients experiencing difficulty in adapting to their heart attacks was made using group psychotherapy. Their wives met for parallel group therapy on alternate weeks. Results indicated patients and their wives appeared to achieve an improved psychosocial adaptation.

3. Altschule M. Updating the cholesterol-atherosclerosis controversy. Primary Care, 1:253-262, June 1974. Very interesting article describing the research that has been done linking the various risk factors to the development of atherosclerosis. Risk factors discussed included dietary intake of cholesterol, hypertension, heredity, diabetes, and smoking. The question of why cholesterol is deposited in the atherosclerotic plaque remains unanswered.

4. Astor S. The road back: cardiac rehabilitation. The Journal of C. V and Pulmonary Technology (reprint) September-December 1973. Excellent article describing, in detail, cardiac rehabilitation programs throughout the country. Topics discussed included functioning of the programs, psychology, group dynamics and home training.

5. Baden C. Pointers coronary patients have given me for improving their care. Consultant, 45-48, July-August, 1968. Excellent article which should be reviewed yearly by CCU nurses. The technique of interviewing former CCU patients is used to improve patient care.

6. Ballantyne DJ. CCTV for patients, American Journal of Nursing, 74:2, 263-264, February, 1974. Description of how one hospital teamed up with a local TV station to produce educational programs for patients. The programs were then shown on closed circuit TV.

7. Berni R, Nicholson C. The POR as a tool in rehabilitation and patient teaching, Nursing Clinics of NA, 9:2, 265-270, June, 1974. A case history is presented to show how the system of problem-oriented charting is utilized in patient teaching.

8. Bessinger H. Physiology of the ischemic heart. Hospital Topics, 44-48, November, 1966. Excellent concise review of cardiovascular physiology.

9. Bille D. The role of body image in patient compliance and education. Heart and Lung, 6:1, 143-148, January-February, 1977. Description of an interesting research project attempting to correlate a positive self-concept with (1) learning during a patient education program, and (2) compliance with prescribed medical regimen following an MI.

10. Bilodeau C, Hackett T. Issues raised in a group setting by patients recovering from myocardial infarction, American Journal of Psychiatry, 128:1 105-109, July, 1971. A "heart club" of five convalescent male cardiac patients met for twelve weeks with an RN who acted as group leader for problem-solving discussions. The issues raised most frequently and suggestions for the discharge planning of similar patients are presented.

11. Bracke NB et al: Patient education by videotape after myocardial infarction: an empirical evaluation. Archives of Physiology and Medical

Rehabilitation, 58:213-219, May, 1977. Very interesting article comparing two methods (videotape and lecture) of presenting educational programs to MI patients. It was shown that completion of a program was more likely to occur when presented on videotape. Other advantages of videotape presentations are cited. (Bibliography of 24)

12. Briant N. When you make your own tape. The Canadian Nurse, 70:12, 38-39, December, 1974. Some pointers, problems and advantages of making your own audiotapes for patient education are explained.

13. Bryan ME. Every nurse a teacher. Annals of Nursing, 4:1, 31-33, July, 1974. Thought-provoking article reviewing the social and cultural influences on the attitudes, beliefs, and learning behaviors of the patient as well as the nurse. The importance of identifying the patient's (rather than the nurse's) needs is stressed.

14. Caplan RM. Educating your patient. Archives of Dermatology, 107: 837-839, June, 1973. Patient education is necessary if we expect compliance with medical therapy. Situations are cited in which more automated information transfer is useful.

15. Douglas JE, Wilkes, TD. Reconditioning cardiac patients. Practical Therapeutics, 11:1, 123-129, Jan. 1975. The benefits of an individualized physical exercise program for the post MI patient are discussed. It is emphasized that this program requires patient education in order to obtain optimal results.

16. Fylling CP, Etzwiler, DD. Health education. Hospitals JAHA, 49: 95-98, April 1, 1975. The need for patient education is stressed. A brief overview of educational programs which have been implemented throughout the country is presented.

17. Gillum RL. Patient education. Journal of the National Medical Association, 66:2, 156-159, March 1974. Excellent article describing the need for education in relation to patient compliance with medical therapy. Individual instruction is cited as the mainstay of patient education. Effectiveness of education can be increased by eliminating barriers to communication.

18. Hackett TP, Cassem NJ. The myocardial infarction patient. Basic Psychiatry for the Primary Care Physician. Boston, Little, Brown and

Co, 1976. Excellent reference for all CCU and cardiac rehabilitation personnel. This chapter explains in detail the psychological responses of an MI patient, beginning with the onset of chest pain through convalescence. Suggestions for appropriate intervention, stressing prevention of anxiety and depression, are detailed.

19. Haldeman J, Thomas P. Classes for coronary care patients. Perspectives in Practice, 63:648-649, December, 1973. Seven principles of dietary teaching for cardiac patients are defined.

20. Hazeltine LS. MI — the weeks of healing, Amercan Journal of Nursing, 64:11 C14-20, November, 1964. Good article describing patient problems and related nursing care in the weeks following an MI. Guidelines to complications, clinical factors and nursing care are listed. Information about anticoagulant therapy is included.

21. Jinks M. The hospital pharmacist in an interdisciplinary inpatient teaching program, American Journal of Hospital Pharmacy, 31:569-574, June, 1974. The pharmacist's involvement in a hospital education program for cardiac patients is described. Specific examples of content, objectives, and patient hand-out materials are presented.

22. Kelsey H, Beamer V. A post-hospital health education program. Heart and Lung, 2:4 512-514, July-August, 1973. The establishment of "Community Heart Clubs" for the education of pre- and post-MI patients are discussed. Problem solving is emphasized to enhance rehabilitation and prevent further illness. The advantages of group therapy are presented.

23. Kinlein ML. MI — the critical hours, American Journal of Nursing, 64:11, C10-13, November, 1964. Excellent article describing the most helpful attitudes and actions a nurse can adopt in caring for a patient in the first few hours following an MI.

24. Knowles MS. Gearing adult education for the seventies. The Journal of Continuing Education in Nursing, 1:1, 11-16, May, 1970. The two major theories of adult learning, behaviorist and humanist, are discussed. The differences between child and adult learning behavior are related to differences in experience and orientation to learning.

25. Krysan GS. Programmed self-instruction: its use in patient education. American Nursing Association Clinical Sessions, San Francisco, Apple-

ton-Century-Crofts, 172-177, 1967. An evaluation of the two types of programmed instruction (linear and branching) as a supplement to the education of adult and child diabetics was performed. The potential for programmed instruction as an educational tool is emphasized.

26. Kucha D. Assessing their needs. Supervisor Nurse, 26-35, April 1974. The author outlines a systematic approach to evaluating the need for patient education programs in outpatient clinincs. Included in the discussion of how to perform a **needs** assessment are the following topics: preparation for analysis, conducting the analysis and methods. The author concludes that a combination of methods is best since this provides cross-checks on the information collected by each means.

27. Lee R, Ball R. Some thoughts on the psychology of the CCU patient, American Journal of Nursing, 75:9, 1498-1505, September, 1975. The various coping responses of MI patients are identified. Response depends on the patient's previous style of adjustment. Suggestions are given for individualizing patient care to enhance optimal adjustment.

28. Lindeman CA. Education and the Hospital, Hospitals, 47: 129-130, March 1, 1973. A short discussion regarding the problems of patient education is presented and one solution to these problems is suggested: creation of sound-on-slide programs by the staff.

29. Moody GC, Duncan JM, Grandbouche A. A program for the teaching of cardiovascular patients. Heart and Lung, 2:4, 508-511, July-August, 1973. The team approach used in this hospital for teaching cardiovascular patients is described. Information given includes: objectives, goals, content, who teaches, audiovisuals used, and patient and physician response to the program.

30. Muller RD. Health education for heart patients in crisis. Health Services Reports, 88:7, 669-675, August-September, 1973. A field research approach emphasizing in-depth interviewing, observation and document reviews, was used to determine the educational needs of the cardiac patient and his family. It is felt that an educational program increases the effectiveness of the process of recovery and prevention of recurrence.

31. Pearson B. Learning tool selection. Supervisor Nurse, 30-31, 1975. Seven general considerations for selecting any patient teaching materials are described.

32. Neeman RL, Neeman M. Complexities of smoking education. The Journal of School Health, 45:1, 17-23, January, 1975. The problems of anti-smoking programs are outlined, but no new solutions are suggested.

33. Rabkin MT. The needs of patients, New England Journal of Medicine, 288-19, 1019-1020, May 10, 1973. A unique telephone hot-line for hospitalized patients is described. Callers receive prompt attention for nonmedical and nonnursing matters having to do with comfort and convenience. The patient's definition of needs as applied to the quality of care is thus considered.

34. Reader G, Schwartz D. Developing patient's knowledge of health. Hospitals, 47: 111-114, March 1, 1973. The need to utilize the patient's in-hospital time for health education purposes is emphasized. Assessing the patient's level of knowledge as part of his medical history.is advocated as is development and follow-up of a long-term health education plan.

35. Redman BK. Guidelines for quality of care in patient education. The Canadian Nurse, 71:19-21, February, 1975. Patient education is defined, process criteria suggested and a priority system for meeting patient's needs is outlined.

36. Redman BK. The Process of Patient Teaching in Nursing, 3rd edition, St. Louis, 1976, The CV Mosby Co.

37. Royle J. Coronary patients and their families receive incomplete care. The Canadian Nurse, 21-25, February, 1973. Excellent article describing the needs of patients at different stages of adaptation following an MI. Suggestions are given for improving care regarding teaching.

38. Rumbaugh DM. The psychological aspects, Journal of Rehabilitation, 56-58, March-April, 1966. Beginning attempts are made to objectively relate psychological factors to the work potential of the cardiac patient.

39.   Skillern RG.   A planned system of patient education, Journal of American Medical Association, 238: 8, 878-879, August 22, 1977. A planned system of patient education featuring (1) a patient education center; (2) a patient educator; and (3) patient education programs is currently in use in group clinics, hospitals and other health care institutions. How the system was established, how it is paid for, its advantages and patient/physician responses are detailed.

40.   Tyzenhouse R.   Myocardial infarction: its effect on the family, American Journal of Nursing, 73: 6, 1012-1013, June, 1973. Small study done by interviewing wives of post-MI patients to determine the family's reactions to the wives who had the most knowledge about the illness and its treatment would have husbands who showed the most progress. This was proved incorrect and it was concluded that the patient should be educated and assume the responsibility for following prescribed therapy.

41.   Ulrich M, Kelley KM. Patient care includes teaching. Hospitals, 46: 59-65, April 1972. Excellent definition of patient education included in this reference.

42.   Weinberg SL. Patient education as part of critical care. Heart and Lung, 3:1 47-48, January-February, 1974. A plea is made for patient education to be considered an essential component of critical care. It is felt that many complications and rehospitalizations of the post-MI patient could be avoided.

43.   Wells C.   Rehabilitation counseling of the heart patient in an outpatient rehabilitation center. Heart and Lung, 3:4, 594-599, July-August, 1974. Excellent discussion of vocational rehabilitation counseling of the cardiac patient. Early intervention by the counselor has proved beneficial to both the patient and the employer.

Postsurgical Conditioning

Sheila Coonen, RN, CVS

In order for a postvascular surgical patient to begin a conditioning program, it is imperative for him to have a complete evaluation to determine any problems he might have that would contraindicate exercise at that particular time, such as congestive heart failure or tachyarrhythmias. This evaluation should include:

1. A complete medical history

2. Physical examination

3. Electrocardiogram

4. Blood and urine analyses (fasting blood glucose, cholesterol, triglyceride concentrations are recommended but not essential)

5. Resting blood pressure

6. A graded, ECG-monitored exercise test (unless medically contraindicated)

For the symptom-limited stress test, we use the United States Air Force protocol (USAFSAM) shown in Table 4.2. It was chosen for its increments of increasing work load per stage, measured in mets (units of metabolic heat production). Using even met increments is important when writing an accurate exercise prescription.

In the Air Force protocol, a person walks at a constant speed of 3.3 mph on a treadmill. The evaluation or grade of the treadmill is increased every three minutes until the person cannot continue to walk. The more common reasons for stopping an exercise test are chest pain, exhaustion, shortness of breath, leg pain, ST segment depression/elevation, and arrhythmias. People being evaluated prior to a conditioning program usually stop walking because of exhaustion, shortness of breath, or leg pain; these are normal responses for a person who is not in good condition. Figure 4.1 shows the results of a typical exercise test using the USAFSAM protocol.

After the physician has interpreted the stress test and found no contraindications to exercise, an exercise prescription can be calculated according to the maximum met level the individual attained during testing. The equations below are used by the American College of Sports Medicine to determine a maximum met level from the percentage of grade and speed of the treadmill.

TABLE 4.2

USAFSAM Protocol

Stage	Speed	Grade	Time	Cum. Time	Mets	Diff/ Stage
6	3.3	25	3	18	14.6	
						2.2
5	3.3	20	3	15	12.4	
						2.2
4	3.3	15	3	12	10.2	
						2.3
3	3.3	10	3	9	7.9	
						2.2
2	3.3	5	3	6	5.7	
						2.2
1	3.3	O	3	3	3.5	

CONVERSION OF GRADE AND SPEED
TO MET LEVELS (WALKING)

Step 1: mph/0.038 = meters/min (m/min)

Step 2: horizontal component = (m/min X 0.1) + 3.5 = maximum oxygen uptake (V_{O_2}) horizontal

Step 3: vertical component = % grade X m/min X 1.8 = maximum oxygen uptake (V_{O_2}) vertical

Step 4: $(V_{O_2}$ horizontal + V_{O_2} vertical)/3.5 = mets

To determine the running met level, substitute 0.2 for 0.1 in step 2.

Once a maximum met level has been determined, a *target* met level must be established. The exercise physiologist must remember that the capacity for performing routine or conditioning work is relatively less in persons with low-function capabilities (six mets or less) than in those with higher inherent capabilities. Cardiac patients are usually able to work at 70% of their maximum, while healthy adults can safely function to 80% to 90% of their maximum met level.

ARIZONA HEART INSTITUTE

Name _Fitt, Jim_

Date _Nov. 2, 1977_

Age _43_ years

Sex _M_

Height _5_ ft. _10_ in.

Weight _173_ lbs.

Tread No. _CT-7246_

Type:
Bruce-------------------1
Blake-------------------2
Bicycle-----------------3
USAFSAM----------------④ MPH _3.3_

Resting ECG:
Normal------------⓪
Myocardial Infarction
  Definite---------1
  Possible---------2
  Location(s)-------
  _____
  _____

Conduction defect--3
  RBBB _____
  LBBB _____
  Other _____

Arrhythmia---------4
  Type _____
  _____

ST Changes---------5
  Elevation _____
  Depression _____
  Nonspecific _____
  Type _____
  _____

L.V. Hypertrophy----6
R.V. Hypertrophy----7
Other _____
  _____
  _____
  _____

Cardiac Medications:
None _____ 1
Pronestyl _____ 2
Quinidine _____ 3
Inderal _____ 4
Digitalis _____ 5
Dilantin _____ 6
Diuretics _____ ⑦
Antihypertensives ____ ⑧
Antidepressants _____ 9
Nitrates _____ ⑩
Potassium _____ 11
Premarin _____ 12
Other _____
  _____
  _____

Indications:
Asymptomatic------------0
Abnormal ECG------------1
Enlarged heart----------2
Atypical chest pain-----3
Stable angina-----------4
Unstable angina---------5
Postinf. angina---------6
Prinzmetal angina-------7
Myocard. Infarction-----8
Heart failure-----------9
Valvular disease-------10
Metabolic disease------11
Conditioning program--⑫
Other _____
  _____
  _____
  _____

Physician _Kinard_

Stage	Time	Heart Rate	Blood Pressure
Rest Supine		96	130/72
I	3	122	172/80
II	6	138	180/70
III	9	160	184/80
IV	12	176	230/80
V			
VI			
VII			
Imm		179	214/78
2MPE		122	148/70
4MPE		124	144/78
6MPE		112	136/70

Comments:

ST-T Wave Changes:
None ___ ☒ 0
I ____
II ____
III ____
AVR ____
AVL ____
AVF ____
V1 ____
V2 ____
V3 ____
V4 ____
V5 ____
V6 ____
J-pt ____

Reason for stopping:
Chest pain------------------1
Exhaustion------------------②
Shortness of breath---------3
Leg pain--------------------4
ST-T depr or elev-----------5
Arrhythmia------------------6

Inability to walk-----------7
Technical reason------------8
Dizziness-------------------9
Blood pressure change------10
Adequate rate response-----11
Other----------------------
  _____
  _____

Interpretation:
Submaximal test-------------1
Inadeq. rate response-------2
ST depr with Digitalis------3
No ischemic changes---------④
ECG changes suggestive of
  ischemia------------------5
Other _____

Figure 4.1. Results of a typical exercise test based upon the USAFSAM protocol.

103

The next question that comes to mind is how can one determine when a person is working at 70%, 80% or 90% of his maximum? This can be ascertained by calculating the person's target heart rate for that percentage of his maximum met level.

CONVERSION OF MET LEVEL TO HEART RATE

Step 1:   [(maximum met level + 60) ÷ 100] x maximum met= target met level

Step 2:   (maximum heart rate* – resting heart rate) X 0.77 + resting heart rate = target heart rate (per min)

*attained during stress testing

Now that a target met level and target heart rate have been established, I recommend a prescription advocated by the American College of Sports Medicine: "An adequate conditioning response can be elicited by maintaining a prescribed work intensity, or a prescribed heart rate, for a period of about fifteen minutes per exercise session. With the inclusion of the important warm-up and cool-down periods, the total duration per session would usually run up to 25 to 30 minutes." They also recommend that exercise sessions be conducted a minimum of three days per week. A typical exercise prescription is shown in Figure 4.2.

At the Arizona Heart Institute, our problem begins by monitoring blood pressure, resting heart rate, and weight. For accuracy in measurement, a 10-sec heart rate is used for both the resting and target rates. Each individual begins his session with warm-up exercises (Figure 4.3). These exercises are listed according to counts per minute and met levels. Each exercise is done for 30 sec, and the number of exercises in the series is determined by the individual's target met level.

Once a target heart rate is reached, the person maintains it for 15 to 25 min by walking, jogging, bike riding, or stair climbing. When the aerobic portion of the exercise session is over, 5 to 10 min are spent doing stretching and relaxation exercises. Each patient is admonished to remain in the laboratory until his heart rate returns to his preexercise resting heart rate, usually 10 minutes. If any individual feels dizzy or nauseated, he is watched carefully until these signs of overexertion subside. Remote telemetry monitoring by electrocardiogram is done weekly or as needed.

In addition to our conditioning personnel of one physician, one nurse, a technician, exercise physiologist, and recreation director, we also have a stress counselor, a dietician, and a vocational rehabilitation counselor. Many of our patients benefit from the services of these counselors.

ARIZONA HEART INSTITUTE

CARDIOVASCULAR CONDITIONING PROGRAM

Exercise Prescription

Name: *Fitt, Jim* Age: *43* Wt: *173* Date: *Nov. 2, 1977*

ETT Results:

Resting HR *96* Resting BP *130/72*

Maximum HR *179* Maximum BP *230/80*

Maximum Met Level *12.5*

Diagnosis: *CORONARY ARTERY DISEASE*

Exercise Prescription:

Target Met Level *8.75*

Target 10 sec. HR *25*

Calesthenics *1 - 14*

Walk: Jog Ratio

_____Walk *All* Jog *147 meters per minute.* Speed

Treadmill _____ *3* MPH *14* %Grade *15 minutes* Time

Volleyball

_____Non-Competitive *✓* Competitive

Jump Rope / Bicycle

Bicycle:

3.2 Kp at 50 strikes per minute

_____*2* Minutes on _____ */* Rest _____ *2* Repetitions

Steps:

20 cm Height *37* Steps/min. *4 minutes* Time

Cool Down

Light weights and stretches

Comments:

Figure 4.2. A sample exercise prescription from the Conditioning Laboratory of the Arizona Heart Institute.

Group exercise sessions have been reported by many to have more than just physical benefits. We have ourselves noted significant psychological improvements with exercise. There are many positive aspects to the feeling of fellowship which develops among people who have experienced the same operation.

By the time each patient has completed two months in the cardiovascular conditioning program, he has been reevaluated and stress tested three times. He may then enter our maintenance program or continue on a home program which we write for him. Every patient is retested six months after

105

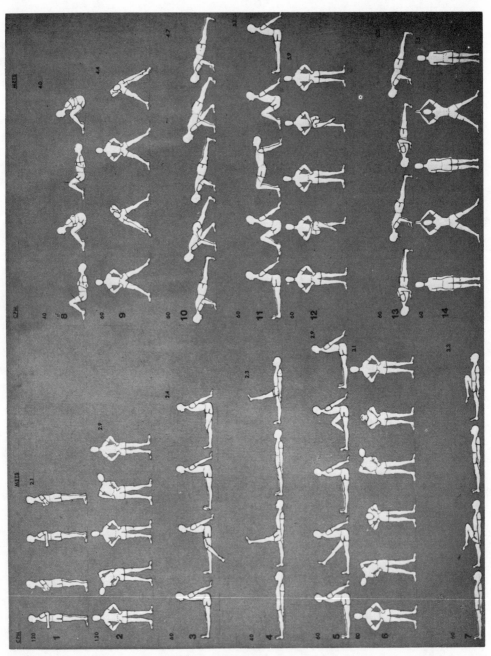

Figure 4.3.   Graded series of exercises used in warm-up session. Each exercise is rated for its met level and the number of counts per minute to attain that level.

completing the program and then yearly thereafter. If, on a return visit, the patient does not surpass his previous exercise level, a not-too-severe reprimand is given, along with a new home exercise prescription! Motivation is extremely important throughout the entire program, and we are continually striving to reinforce a patient's sense of well being and self-confidence so that he will continue his exercise program.

REFERENCES

1. American College of Sports Medicine, Guidelines for Graded Exercise Testing and Exercise Prescription, Philadelphia, Lea & Febiger, 1976.

2. American College of Sports Medicine, Handout (meeting in LaCrosse, Wisconsin), 1976.

3. Committee on Exercise, Exercise Testing and Training of Apparently Healthy Individuals: A Handbook for Physicians, New York, American Heart Association, 1972.

4. Committee on Exercise, Exercise Testing and Training of Individuals with Heart Disease or at High Risk for Its Development: A Handbook for Physicians, Dallas, American Heart Association, 1975.

5. Dill DB. Oxygen used in horizontal and grade walking and running on the treadmill. J App Physiol, 20:19-22, 1965.

6. Ellestad MH. Stress Testing, Philadelphia, FA Davis, 1975.

7. Margaria R. Energy cost of running. J Appl Physiol, 18: 367-70, 1962. 1962.

8. Naughton J, Hellerstein H. Exercise Testing and Exercise Training in Coronary Heart Disease, New York, Academic Press, 1973.

9. Weis R, Karpovich P. Energy cost for exercise for convalescents. Arch Phy Med 26: 447-54, 1947.

Section 5
Myocardial Preservation

Nurses associated with cardiovascular medicine should be aware of some of the major research areas in this rapidly changing field. At the moment, myocardial preservation, the protection of myocardial cells from hypoxic damage, is in the forefront of cardiovascular research. Injury to the myocardium during cardiac surgery is to some extent unavoidable. Organs must be retracted, muscles divided, arteries ligated. These traumatic aspects of surgery are inescapable at the level of our technological development today. However, interference in the metabolism of the cells composing the heart is a complication of our refined technology. Extracorporeal circulation and aortic cross-clamping are both highly valuable techniques in cardiac surgery, but they interrupt the oxygen supply to the cardiac muscle by shutting off the blood. In a heart that has already suffered similar damage due to ischemia, the resultant insult to the myocardium could be injurious or even fatal. Hence, cardiovascular surgeons are now looking for a way to eliminate these adverse effects of modern surgical technique.

The following paper presents a review of the evolution of the myocardial preservation theory and the techniques used in the last decade. Further, it provides an instructional section on cardiac cellular metabolism which will help to explain the damage hypoxia can cause and the metabolic standards which an effective myocardial preservation technique must meet.

Myocardial Preservation
A Historical and Biochemical Review

Edward B. Diethrich, MD

One of the most current and intensely researched issues in cardiovascular surgery is the problem of myocardial preservation during cardiac surgery. For over two decades, open heart surgery has been performed, and in that time, numerous operative and ancillary techniques have been developed only to fall by the wayside as research and innovation introduced technological improvements. Myocardial preservation is now one of these rapidly evolving methodologies.

As operative procedures become more involved, and the periods of extracorporeal circulation and aortic cross-clamping are extended, the myocardium is increasingly likely to sustain permanent damage. Experimental studies have shown that potentially irreversible, identifiable metabolic and structural lesions occur in the myocardium after only 10 minutes of induced ischemia. Although hypoxia is an adverse effect of aortic cross-clamping, the advantages of this technique make it desirable, for the moment at least. Hence, cardiovascular surgeons at the Arizona Heart Institute have turned their attention to refining both the theory and technique of myocardial preservation in an effort to reduce this hypoxic damage.

MYOCARDIAL PRESERVATION – GOALS AND TECHNIQUES

No one will deny that surgery is a traumatic experience, both emotionally and physically. However, the potential lifesaving benefits generally outweigh the deleterious consequences. In cardiovascular surgery, one of the major problems is irreversible myocardial damage resulting from hypoxia.

Theoretically, myocardial preservation seeks to obviate the insidious effects of surgically-related hypoxia. In translating this theory into a workable technique, optimum protection has been associated with three goals: 1) to minimize myocardial injury; 2) to permit maximum operative exposure; and 3) to ensure a quiet operative field.

Both aortic cross-clamping and cardiopulmonary bypass have been relatively successful in satisfying the second and third goals by producing a still, bloodless field. However, they cause hypoxidosis and its resultant cellular damage. Moreover, coronary self-perfusion, even after clamping the aorta, is often sufficient to maintain the heart's pumping action unless complete left ventricular venting is accomplished. An ideal myocardial preservation technique should solve all these problems.

Members of our staff have been studying myocardial protective methods for over ten years, having begun during the cardiac transplantation era. At that time, viable hearts were isolated *in vivo* with a fixed amount of blood in them by ligating the thoracic aorta, the aortic arch branch vessels, and the *vena cavae*. The hearts were then removed to preservation chambers in which they were perfused with an oxygenated solution of nutrients. The hearts continued to beat with good myocardial function for up to 44 hours. Histologic examination of the myocardium after preservation (Figure 5.1) showed no damage to the cells as a result of extracorporeal preservation.

Experiments such as these paved the way for future intraoperative studies of myocardial preservation. Over the intervening years, many techniques have been devised to provide the optimum conditions for operative exposure with minimum myocardial insult: ischemic arrest, continuous cardiac pumping, systemic hypothermia, ventricular fibrillation, pericardial

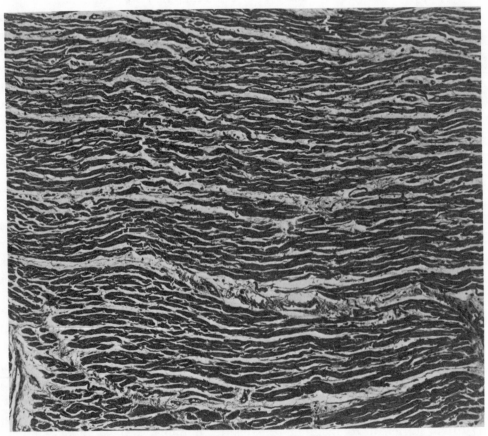

Figure 5.1   Myocardial tissue from a heart preserved 44 hours extracorporeally showing normal cellular structure (H&E,x46.8)

slush, and potassium arrest. But none of these methods has proven entirely satisfactory. Ischemic arrest produces cellular injury within 10 minutes at normal body temperatures, so it is not applicable to most current cardio-vascular operations. Working on a continuously beating heart, especially during aortocoronary bypass procedures, makes performance of the distal anastomosis quite difficult. Systemic hypothermia was a significant advancement in the area of myocardial protection, but alone, it does not provide optimum pro-tection for prolonged periods of time. Nonetheless, hypothermia is a vital *part* of currently used protective measures. Ventricular fibrillation is a particularly disadvantageous technique, since the fibrillating heart uses a significant amount of energy, thereby compromising the myocardium.

Pericardial slush enjoyed a brief surge of popularity recently, since a locally hypothermic response was thought to produce further decreases in metabolic rate. However, we performed a study of this technique measuring myocardial temperatures at the epicardial, midcardiac, and intracardiac sur-faces in four locations around the heart. By way of contrast, the same protocol was applied to the cardioplegic technique. It was found that the pericardial slush cooled only the epicardium, while cardioplegia achieved more uniform cooling throughout the layers of the myocardium.

Potassium arrest, like hypothermia, has now become a valuable part of the myocardial preservation technique. Originally, it was used some 20 years ago to interrupt heart action, but its use was discontinued due to tox-icity problems.

From all these investigations and trials certain key components of the ideal myocardial preservation technique could be identified. First among these is hypothermia. Lowering tissue temperature decreases the metabolic rate. Minimal intracardiac blood volume is also important to prevent cardiac disten-tion. Intracardiac pressure increases when the heart becomes overfilled with blood, and this contributes to an elevation of intramyocardial pressure with resultant cellular damage. Acid-base balance and electrolyte balance are two obviously vital principles to which attention must be paid. Lastly, and prob-ably most significantly, we have cellular nourishment or substrate enhance-ment. Early cardiac preservation protocols employed insulin and glucose in the perfusion solution; today, we find we are returning to some of this old knowledge to preserve the myocardium *in vivo*.

MYOCARDIAL METABOLISM

The myocardial cell, or myofiber, is distinguishable from other types of mammalian muscle in its intrinsic ability to depolarize all its components simultaneously, causing it to beat synchronously. This and other special properties of the myofiber are the result of cellular specialization. That is, myocardial cells with the same fundamental anatomic construction assume one task or function, thereby developing different electrophysiological characteristics. Essentially, though, there are two *functional* types — cells which generate or propogate exciting impulses and ones which produce the contractile force.

Our discussion will center now around myocardial metabolism, which is similar for all myofibers, but first we must identify the major components of the cell. Figure 5.2 is a representation of a group of myocardial cells. The cell membrane, or sarcolemma, sustains excitation and couples it to contraction. In some myofibers, the sarcolemma permeates the cell's interior sarcoplasm with a system of tubules known as the T-system (transverse tubular system). Since this T-system is contiguous with the sarcolemma, it effectively expands the surface membrane, enlarging the pathway for the electrical impulses which induce contraction.

Within the cell are the sarcomeres arranged in myofibrils, long rows running the length of the cell. The bulk of the cell is composed of these contractile units, which are activated by calcium ion transport. Intimately surrounding these myofibrils is an intricately branching tubule system called the sarcoplasmic retriculum. After the contractive event has begun and the calcium

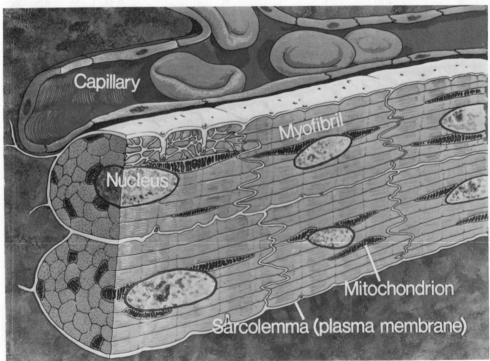

Figure 5.2   Representation of a group of normal myocardial cells.

114

ion concentration increases to stimulate the sarcomeres, the sarcoplasmic reticulum is activated to pump the cation away from the myofibrils, stopping contraction and producing relaxation. In short then, electrical impulses originating at the atrioventricular node pass along the sarcolemma and its T-system, producing calcium ion transport to the sarcomeres. Thus stimulated, the sarcomeres contract in proportion to the cation concentration. When this concentration reaches a near critical point (one at which the sarcomeres would be irreversibly contracted), the sarcoplasmic reticulum funnels the calcium away from the sarcomeres to holding areas in the cytoplasm. Contraction ceases, the sarcomeres relax, and the entire event is ready to be repeated.

The nucleus and mitochondria, the other major elements of the cell, are engaged in cell maintenance and energy production. The centrally located nucleus is the repository for the genetically coded ribonucleic acid, which is required for growth, maintenance, and repair. The large elliptical mitochondrial bodies, lying in close proximity to the sarcomeres, contain the complex elements necessary for oxidative phosphorylation, the energy producing process within the cell. Since this is the site of energy generation in the cell, it is to this structure that we look to examine the efficacy of preservation techniques.

Now that the cellular components of the myofiber have been explained functionally, the next step is to understand myocardial metabolism. Cardiac metabolism is unique because it must produce energy constantly in a highly efficient manner to supply the continuously beating heart. Hence, the myocardium metabolizes glucose, its preferred substrate, aerobically, by far a more efficient method than anaerobic metabolism. In time of nutritional deprivation, the heart can resort to anaerobic metabolism to maintain life, but there are two more preferable alternate energy sources in the cell, fatty acids and stored glycogen, a polymer of glucose.

During energy production, the cell must metabolize its nutrients at a nearly constant temperature to maintain cellular integrity. This can be accomplished only by multiple stage oxidations which transform substrate into carbon dioxide and water. During this sequence of oxidations, electrons are released to be transported by coenzymes in the "electron transfer chain." At each transfer point in the chain, energy is generated and used to produce ATP, the prime energy source for the cell by virtue of its terminal high energy phosphate bond. This entire series of reactions culminating in the production of ATP is called oxidative phosphorylation.

To illustrate this more specifically, a mole of glucose can be followed through the entire metabolic process (Figure 5.3). In the cytoplasm, glucose is broken down to pyruvic acid through decarboxylation and dehydrogenation. This pyruvic acid is transported to the mitochondria where it enters the regenerating citric acid (Kreb's) cycle. Prior to entering the cycle, the pyruvate is transformed into acetyl coenzyme A, a vital component in metabolism. This

Metabolism of Glucose

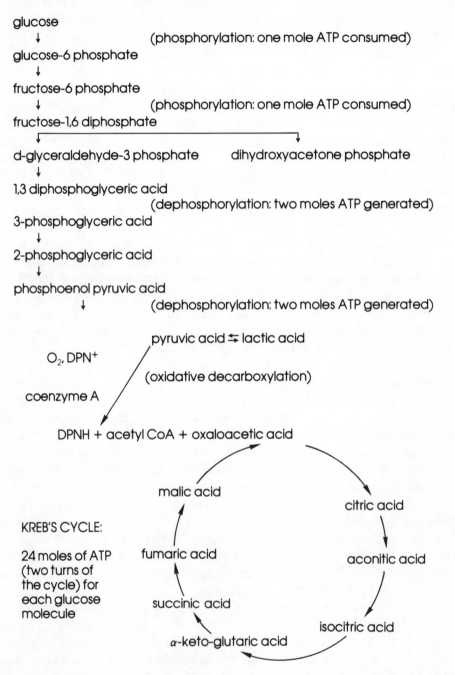

glucose
↓ (phosphorylation: one mole ATP consumed)
glucose-6 phosphate
↓
fructose-6 phosphate
↓ (phosphorylation: one mole ATP consumed)
fructose-1,6 diphosphate

d-glyceraldehyde-3 phosphate   dihydroxyacetone phosphate
↓
1,3 diphosphoglyceric acid
(dephosphorylation: two moles ATP generated)
3-phosphoglyceric acid
↓
2-phosphoglyceric acid
↓
phosphoenol pyruvic acid
↓ (dephosphorylation: two moles ATP generated)

pyruvic acid ⇄ lactic acid

O_2, DPN⁺

(oxidative decarboxylation)

coenzyme A

DPNH + acetyl CoA + oxaloacetic acid

malic acid

citric acid

KREB'S CYCLE:

24 moles of ATP
(two turns of
the cycle) for
each glucose
molecule

fumaric acid

aconitic acid

succinic acid

isocitric acid

α-keto-glutaric acid

Figure 5.3   The oxidative phosphorylation sequence and Kreb's (citric acid) cycle.

116

coenzyme begins the chain reactions which transform it into oxaloacetic acid, producing two moles of CO_2 for each mole of acetyl coenzyme A utilized. This cycle will continue as long as acetyl coenzyme A is available, attesting to the importance of this pyruvic acid derivative.

ATP is generated at three points in this cycle for a total of 12 moles of ATP per mole of acetyl coenzyme A. Since one mole of glucose produces two moles of pyruvic acid, the cycle can turn twice, giving 24 moles of ATP per mole of glucose. But ATP is also produced at the pyruvic acid to acetyl coenzyme A oxidation (6 moles twice) and during the anaerobic metabolism of glucose to pyruvate (2 moles) for a grand total of 38 moles of ATP for each mole of glucose.

In terms of energy units (calories), oxidation of glucose to carbon dioxide and water produces 686 kilocalories. Each mole of ATP requires 8 kilocalories to produce, so there are 304 kilocalories returned to the cell for an efficiency of 45%. By comparison, if the cell had to metabolize pyruvate anaerobically, an efficiency of less than 10% would be realized.

What does all this chemistry have to do with myocardial preservation? Well, it is the knowledge of these intricate chemical processes which supports the rationale for our current myocardial protective techniques. As shown

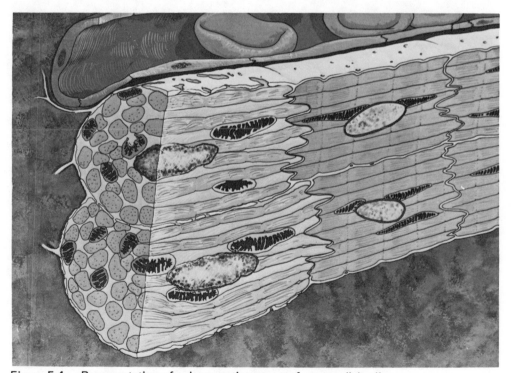

Figure 5.4   Representation of a degenerating group of myocardial cells.

previously, there are certain key compounds which must be present and various structures which must function if the myocardium is to metabolize normally. Normal myocardial function, meeting the demand for energy, is the objective of myocardial preservation. Hence, the preservative technique must provide nutrients and prevent damage to vital structures. If the protective effect fails, the sarcolemma deteriorates, the nuclei begin to clump, the sarcomeres become irregular, and the mitochondria become edematous (Figure 5.4). This mitochondrial swelling leads to vacuolation within the bodies. Figure 5.5 is an electron microscopic picture of a real cell in the final stages of destruction. Note particularly the condition of the mitochondria.

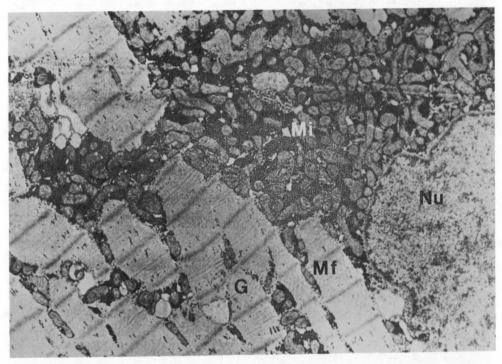

Figure 5.5   Electron micrograph of degenerating myocardial tissue. Notice the small size and number of mitochondria. (Nu = nucleus; Mf = myofibril; G = glycogen granules; Mi = mitochondrion)

Research to discover the ideal method of preserving the myocardial tissue during cardiac surgery is an ongoing effort, and the best we can provide today is an interim solution to the problem. The latest in the line of myocardial protective techniques is hypothermic, pharmacologic cardioplegia. Although several different procedures have been proposed for this technique, we have standardized our method: total cardiopulmonary bypass at 28°C is begun and the ascending aorta cross-clamped. A 15-gauge catheter is inserted in the aorta proximal to the clamp and 350 cc of cold (4°C) cardioplegic solution is rapidly infused under pressure. The infusion cannula is then connected to a suction line for continuous myocardial venting through the aortic valve.

The components of our cardioplegic solution include: Plasmanate, albumin, dextrose, insulin, calcium chloride, tromethamine (THAM), procaine hydrochloride, and potassium chloride. Each of these elements addresses a different area in the metabolic state.

Plasmanate, the volume expanding vehicle for the cardioplegia solution, has a viscosity that closely approximates that of blood and it contains several plasma constituents. Dextrose and insulin provide substrate enhancement, insulin helping to convert dextrose to glycogen for anaerobic metabolism. Albumin renders the solution hyperosmolar to encourage substrate passage into the myofibers.

Both hypothermia and cardiopulmonary bypass induce swelling of the myofiber. When this occurs, water and sodium pass into the cell, potassium exits, and electrolyte imbalance results. Although the solution is made hypertonic to counteract the accumulation of water in the tissues, the calcium ion concentration within the cell is adversely affected by any electrolyte imbalance. Since this one element is vital to proper myocardial contraction, it is imperative that an adequate concentration of calcium exists when the heart resumes beating, hence the addition of calcium chloride.

Metabolic acidosis, precipitated by both hypothermia and aortic cross-clamping, interferes with anaerobic metabolism. In order to counteract this acidosis and maintain a physiologic pH level, the cardioplegic solution is buffered with either THAM (tromethamine) or bicarbonate to a 7.6 pH. To insure the integrity of the cell membrane, various pharmacologic agents may be used to stabilize the sarcolemma against the effects of intracellular swelling. Steroids or procaine hydrochloride may be used for this purpose. Lastly, the potassium is used to induce immediate asystole, sparing the energy reserves of the myofibers.

The single infusion of the cardioplegic solution after cross-clamping will protect the myocardium only as long as the nutrients last and metabolism is retarded by reduced temperatures. Recognizing this deficiency, we have resorted to periodic reinfusion of the cardioplegic solution during the operation to replace substrate, remove metabolites discarded during the anaerobic process, and keep all tissue layers of the heart cold. Moreover, we have learned that areas of the heart fed by stenotic coronary arteries may not be receiving adequate, uniform amounts of the cardioplegic solution through the primary route (ascending aorta). For this reason, we also reinfuse 35 cc aliquots of cardioplegic solution through each aortocoronary bypass vein graft after the distal anastomosis is complete. In this way, myocardial tissue can receive the benefits of the cardioplegic solution via the aorta or, in areas of occluded coronary arteries, through the newly revascularized route.

Continued research will no doubt lead to a better understanding of myocardial metabolism and ultimately the development of a protective technique assuring 100% preservation while providing ideal operating conditions. Even now, another new idea is being considered — the substitution of whole blood as the major transport vehicle, and new pharmacologic agents which directly affect cellular metabolism are approaching clinical trials. So the search goes forward — always striving for a simpler, better method to protect the myocardium from hypoxic damage.

Section 6

Postoperative Complications

Everyone in the medical profession is keenly aware of the unique level of care the surgical patient requires in those first hours and days following surgery. It is at this time that many types of complications may arise which demand prompt recognition and treatment if the patient is to survive. The totally helpless, often noncommunicative, postsurgical patient is placed in the hands of nurses who must be trained to identify signs of impending problems and respond to the situation intelligently and aggressively.

Efforts are being made daily by surgeons and physicians to reduce the likelihood of postoperative complications, but the inherent untoward effects of anesthesia and pharmacological agents alone are responsible for many postsurgical crises. Potential complications arising from the surgical procedure itself, particularly in the cardiac cases employing cardiopulmonary bypass, anticoagulation, and prosthetics, are numerous, although thankfully, not as common today.

The papers in this section address three main areas of postsurgical complications: pulmonary, hematologic, and cardiac. Each of these papers presents a review of the possible complications, their symptoms, and the treatment advised today. Moreover, suggestions are made by the authors for procedures which could reduce the incidence of certain adverse patient response in these three systems.

Postoperative Pulmonary Complications

Robert J. Clark, MD, FACP

Many persons undergo some type of major surgical procedure yearly, and a significant portion have pulmonary disease. Pulmonary complications, defined as respiratory failure, atelectasis, pneumonia, hypoxemia, aspiration, pulmonary embolism, pneumothorax, and secretion retention occur with alarming frequency. If one uses the alveolar-arterial difference in oxygen tension, (A-a) DO_2, almost all postoperative patients suffer from some degree of respiratory embarrassment. The location and type of surgery performed appear to be well correlated with the risk of pulmonary complications. For example, they are more frequent in thoracic and upper abdominal surgery and far less frequent in peripheral surgery. The purpose of this brief discussion is to define the problem, examine the complications, identify the factors which predispose to pulmonary complications, learn their early recognition and diagnosis, perform the necessary treatment, and hopefully find methods of preventing them.

Of the above mentioned respiratory complications, the most common are atelectasis, respiratory failure, secretion retention, and pneumonia. Respiratory failure is defined as any fall in $Pa\,O_2$ or rise of $Pa\,CO_2$ beyond the normal range. The degree of failure and the ultimate treatment depends upon the degree of change, the rate of change, and the duration of the abnormality. We are less concerned with moderate hypoxemia in a patient with long-standing emphysema than we would be in a previously healthy individual.

The key to effective use of a therapeutic armamentarium and hopefully the prevention of pulmonary complications is a good basic foundation consisting of a general history and physical examination of each patient. A general history is essential, but we must emphasize the importance of a detailed pulmonary history. This history must include any smoking exposure, the presence or absence of cough, shortness of breath, dyspnea on exertion, asthma, or allergies. Other factors we must try to identify are preexisting pulmonary infection, emphysema, chronic bronchitis, interstitial fibrosis, previous lung surgery, neuromuscular disease, obesity, kyphoscoliosis, and poor nutritional status. Smoking is the most common cause of chronic bronchitis and emphysema. It is also one of the most important factors which predispose patients to pulmonary complications such as secretion retention and infection following surgery.

Once pulmonary symptoms have been ascertained, more specific questioning and investigation into these symptoms can be performed. The simple presence of a cough or shortness of breath does not necessarily mean that the patient has lung disease because these symptoms are not specific and may represent occult heart disease. The same is true for dyspnea on exertion. The presence of a chronic cough with sputum production present for many years, however, is very typical of chronic bronchitis and does imply pulmonary disease. Slowly progressive shortness of breath in a smoking individual would imply emphysema, but further history and testing is required to identify other diseases such as interstitial fibrosis.

In the asthmatic patient, a careful drug history is required with special emphasis placed on the recent and past use of corticosteroids. Asthmatic patients tend to decompensate under stress of surgery. Previous lung surgery has obvious implications since the removal of lung tissue decreases the individual's pulmonary reserve. Pulmonary reserve is likewise decreased in neuro-muscular disease, kyphoscoliosis, obesity, and poor nutrition. Thoracic and high abdominal incisions markedly reduce the functional reserve of the lung and thereby decrease the flow rates and ability to remove secretions effectively.

Preoperative pulmonary function studies are of value in selected instances. They are useful to detect and quantify chronic obstructive pulmonary disease, interstitial pulmonary fibrosis, and asthma. Many studies have been performed to identify the individual at risk by means of pulmonary function tests. These studies have been contradictory to each other, primarily because of the wide range of variability for each pulmonary function test. It is generally accepted, however, that if the 1 sec forced expiratory volume (FEV_1) is less than 1 liter, or there is significant carbon dioxide retention greater than 50 mm Hg, then pulmonary complications are very likely. This again depends on the type of surgery to be performed, and one might have a separate set of criteria for peripheral surgery and abdominal surgery. Other criteria might be used for pulmonary resection surgery.

Once the individual with factors predisposing him to pulmonary complications has been identified, certain measures can be taken prior to any surgical procedure. The best way to prevent postoperative pulmonary problems is to anticipate them preoperatively. Smoking should be stopped as soon as surgery is contemplated, preferably weeks prior to surgery. Pulmonary infection must be diagnosed accurately and treated vigorously with antibiotic selection dictated by sputum culture and gram stain. Secretions can be controlled with proper humidification and chest physiotherapy. Asthmatics, especially those who have recently received corticosteriod therapy, require frequent assessment of their status, including the effectiveness of bronchodilator therapy. The use of corticosteroids should be considered in a symptomatic asthmatic or in an asthmatic with a history of recent steroid therapy who will soon undergo a surgical procedure. It is also important to familiarize the patient with the methods of treatment to which he will be exposed after surgery. These will include the use of chest physiotherapy, either small volume nebulizer therapy or intermittent positive pressure devices, incentive spirometers, aerosol masks, and effective methods of coughing in the presence of severe pain. In certain individuals, postoperative mechanical ventilation will be necessary and the use of the various mechanical devices should be explained to the patient.

In the immediate postoperative period, dramatic changes have occurred in the respiratory system. Vital capacity has decreased, ciliary function is compromised, the cough reflex is diminished, and fear of pain is present. To either forestall or overcome pulmonary complications, a host of methods, both voluntary and involuntary, have been devised. Most of these are designed to reduce the frequency and magnitude of postoperative atelectasis. Intermittent positive pressure breathing (IPPB) is one of the more widely used treatments. The rationale behind its use is that the positive pressure will expand the lungs to larger volumes and prevent or reverse atelectasis. IPPB must be administered by an experienced therapist who will not only monitor the effectiveness of therapy but also assure that the tidal volume is indeed greater than that which could be achieved spontaneously. It is useful to deliver aerosolized medications, such as bronchodilators, and to temporarily increase minute ventilation. Frequently overlooked, however, are the disadvantages of IPPB therapy, which include possibly no change in tidal volumes unless the patient is coaxed, interference with cardiac venous return, gastric distention, and the risk of infection or cross-contamination from colonized equipment. For effective use, tidal volume must be monitored with each breath to assure that it is greater than that which the patient can inspire voluntarily. In practice, this is rarely done, and the physician, assuming its effectiveness, fails to use other methods of treatment.

In a patient unable to move easily in bed, frequent turning from side to side is important. For the heavily sedated patient with an artificial airway in place, the routine use of frequent turning, along with frequent suctioning, is mandatory. Other methods to be described below are more appropriate for the patient who is able to cooperate with the therapist or nurse.

Voluntary deep breathing is the least expensive mode of therapy, and it can be very effective when inspiration is slow and the breath held temporarily at peak inspiration. No apparatus is needed and the intrapleural pressures are physiologic. Unfortunately, the patient must be very well motivated and highly cooperative.

Blow bottles, once quite popular, are seldom used today. The most beneficial effect is in taking a deep breath prior to displacing the fluid from one container to another. The intra-alveolar pressures are theoretically evenly distributed throughout the lungs, but practically they probably are not. Unfortunately, this technique emphasizes expiration and it is possible that if a patient expires below his functional residual capacity (FRC), he could cause more atelectasis than he originally had. This technique is not recommended for routine use.

The incentive spirometer is a variation of a voluntary deep breathing technique wherein the patient is given an indication of his effort as a "reward." Several types of incentive spirometers are available, and the prices range widely. Two popular examples of incentive spirometer are the Bartlett-Edwards (McGaw) and Triflo (Clinical Products) ball type incentive spirometer. The ball type incentive spirometer is no less effective than the Bartlett-Edwards model and is five to six times less expensive. In addition, the patient is able with various involuntary treatments. Carbon dioxide rebreathing into a one-the hospital. The emphasis is appropriately on inspiration, but cooperation and motivation are required.

The above mentioned methods are voluntary and can be supplemented with various involuntary treatments. Carbon dioxide rebreathing into a one-liter dead space will cause most individuals to increase their minute ventilation. It is an inexpensive and simple technique and can be performed with a minimum of cooperation. Unfortunately, hypercapnia and hypoxemia may result. The hypoxemia may be treated by enriching the mixture with oxygen. The patient, however, may simply increase the rate of respiration and not depth of respiration, especially if pain is involved. If the depth of respiration is not increased, the treatment will be ineffective.

Chest physiotherapy and partial drainage can be utilized effectively to mobilize secretions and promote coughing. It involves a great deal of therapist's time and can be performed only intermittently throughout the day. It is usually quite fatiguing to the patient and can be painful in certain individuals, especially those who have had thoracic surgery. An experienced therapist is required for effective delivery. One of the advantages of this form of therapy is that of stimulating the patient and encouraging him to cough and deep breathe.

Ultrasonic nebulization of water or saline can be irritating to the larynx, upper airway, and cause bronchospasm. Hypertonic saline has also been used. The value of this therapy depends on the effectiveness of the cough reflex which, if absent, will be less valuable except for hydrating secretions. The involuntary cough reflex, hopefully, would cause an involuntary deep inspiration prior to the tussive effort. It is simple to use, but the machines are expensive and require regular scrupulous cleaning to prevent contamination. Tachyphylaxis to the mist may occur.

Nasotracheal suction is frequently used, and in certain instances can be quite helpful. The secretions within the trachea and mainstem bronchi can be removed and stimulate the cough reflex. It is, however, very uncomfortable and requires skill in executing. Sometimes it is very difficult to introduce a

126

catheter into the trachea, and cardiac arrhythmias, hypoxemia, tracheal damage, bronchospasm, or laryngospasm will occur. Percutaneous tracheal catheters are infrequently used, but have the same effect as nasotracheal suction. A solution of saline can be instilled directly into the trachea and stimulate the cough relfex. If the cough reflex is not present, however, this treatment will be ineffective, except to hydrate the secretions.

Therapeutic bronchoscopy is an invaluable tool in the maintenance of airway patency, and can be used in certain individuals with segmental or total lung collapse. It rapidly aids the patient in relieving obstructive secretions, but it is expensive and not without risk. Cardiac arrhythmias, hypoxia, anesthetic reaction, and trauma can occur. It must be performed by a physician experienced in the technique, and is helpful only in conjunction with other types of therapy.

The most serious respiratory complication is the adult respiratory distress syndrome (ARDS) or shock lung. This syndrome is characterized by massive confluent lung infiltrates, a marked decrease in functional residual capacity (FRC), microthrombosis of pulmonary arterioles, pulmonary shuntting, ventilation perfusion abnormalities, infection, increased lung water, and a marked increase in the work of breathing. This syndrome almost invariably requires early intubation and treatment with positive end–expiratory pressure (PEEP). A person requiring mechanical ventilation and artificial airway is exposed to a whole host of other pulmonary complications. The endotracheal tube itself might cause damage to the larynx or the trachea. For this reason, low cuff pressure endotracheal tubes are preferred. The low pressure cuff tends to conform to the irregularities of a trachea rather than have the trachea conform to the balloon of the endotracheal tube. If secretions become a problem or if the ventilatory support will be long term, a tracheostomy should be performed. One must pay careful attention to increases in lung water and treat early. Swan-Ganz catheterization with the measurement of left ventricular end-diastolic pressures and pulmonary artery pressures is useful. Alveolar collapse and decrease in FRC can be prevented and treated by the use of PEEP. PEEP is associated with an increase incidence of pneumothorax, mediastinal and subcutaneous emphysema, and a decreased cardiac output. The benefits of PEEP, however, are usually to lessen the possibility of pulmonary oxygen toxicity by allowing one to use lower concentrations of inspired oxygen. Alveolar collapse may be treated by ventilating the patient with large tidal volumes. Infection must be treated vigorously with appropriate antibiotics in appropriate doses. The mortality of ARDS in a postoperative patient is between 20% and 50%.

In summary, it is best to avoid rather than treat postoperative pulmonary complications. The early recognition and diagnosis of the factors predisposing to respiratory complications by taking a good history and performing a complete physical examination can be very helpful in identifying those individuals who are at great risk. Many types of therapy are available to prevent pulmonary complications, but probably the most important is the cessation of smoking. One must always remember that each type of therapy carries its own risks and complications and must be used judiciously. For most patients with minor complications, the incentive spirometer device is ideal, provided the individuals are well motivated and understand what is required. For those individuals who are unable to cooperate or refuse to do so, one of the other modalities may be used.

REFERENCES

1. Bartlett RH, et al. Respiratory maneuvers to prevent postoperative pulmonary complications. JAMA, 224:1017, 1973.

2. Gold MI. The present status if IPPB therapy. Chest, 67:469, 1975.

3. Murray JF. Review of the state of the art in intermittent positive pressure breathing therapy. Am Rev Resp Dis, 107:193, 1975.

4. Parsons EF, et al. Effect of positive pressure breathing on distribution of pulmonary blood flow and ventilation. Am Rev Resp Dis, 103:356, 1971.

5. Van De Waser JM, et al. Prevention of postoperative pulmonary complications. Surgery, Gynecology & Obstetrics, 135:229, 1972.

Cardiac Arrhythmias

John Stoner, MD

Cardiac arrhythmias occur frequently during open-heart surgery and in the immediate postoperative period. As many forms of heart disease are now amenable to surgery, the full spectrum of rhythm disturbances may be seen. A detailed description of such a broad topic is beyond the scope of this discussion. Rather a general approach to assessing and treating cardiac arrhythmias in the postoperative period will be presented, followed by more specific comments on the arrhythmias most commonly encountered in this setting.

GENERAL APPROACH

In managing any patient with a cardiac arrhythmia, four basic steps should be followed (Table 6.1). First, the arrhythmia must be correctly diagnosed. This relies mainly on the electrocardiogram, though many clues are available from the physical examination.

TABLE 6.1

General Approach to the Management of Cardiac Arrhythmias

1. Correct diagnosis of the arrhythmia (electrocardiogram, physical examination)
2. Search for an underlying cause of the arrhythmia
3. Assessment of the hemodynamic effect of the arrhythmia
4. Institution of therapy (correction of underlying abnormality, antiarrhythmic drugs)

Second, a search should be made for an underlying cause of the arrhythmia. The patient undergoing open-heart surgery obviously has significant cardiac disease and this in itself is frequently the cause. Metabolic derangements and local mechanical or inflammatory processes also commonly underlie arrhythmias during this period.

Third, the hemodynamic effect of the arrhythmia must be assessed. This in turn will dictate how rapidly treatment is to be instituted. Rhythm disturbances which produce a marked reduction in cardiac output and profound hypotension obviously must be treated immediately, while those that produce little hemodynamic change may be managed best conservatively with a period of observation before instituting therapy. During this time the rhythm disturbance may resolve spontaneously.

Finally, after following these first three steps, the appropriate treatment must be chosen based upon the type of arrhythmia and its underlying cause, the rapidity with which it is instituted being dictated by the patient's hemodynamic status. Treatment may involve specific measures to correct underlying metabolic problems or the use of antiarrhythmic drugs.

ETIOLOGY OF ARRHYTHMIAS

The postoperative cardiac patient presents a very complex picture in which many factors may interplay to predispose to arrhythmias (Table 6.2).

TABLE 6.2

Etiology of Arrhythmias Following Cardiac Surgery

1. Nature and severity of underlying cardiac disease
2. Anesthesia
3. Surgical manipulation or injury
4. Hypothermia
5. Metabolic abnormalities
6. Pericardial disease
7. Drug toxicity

1. The underlying cardiac abnormality for which surgery was performed is probably the most important factor. Certain forms of heart disease are frequently associated with specific types of arrhythmias which persist or recur in the postoperative period.

Among patients with congenital heart disease, atrial arrhythmias are commonly encountered. Examples include atrial septal defect, Ebstein's anomaly, and tricuspid atresia, all of which are frequently associated with atrial fibrillation. In valvular heart disease, atrial arrhythmias and conduction abnormalities may be seen. Mitral valve stenosis or regurgitation produces left atrial enlargement which in turn predisposes to to atrial fibrillation. Calcific aortic stenosis in elderly patients may be associated with conduction system disease that can progress to complete heart block postoperatively. Patients with coronary artery disease undergoing saphenous vein bypass graft surgery are more likely to develop premature ventricular contractions, ventricular tachycardia, or fibrillation.

Not only the nature, but the severity, of the underlying cardiac abnormality is important in the development of postoperative arrhythmias. Patients in functional class III or IV are more likely to have significant cardiac arrhythmias than those with milder disease and are more likely to die as a result of them.

2. Anesthetic agents may predispose to cardiac arrhythmias, both directly through toxic effects on cardiac tissue, and indirectly by sensitizing the heart to the effects of catecholamines. Catecholamine blood levels increase in response to the stress of open-heart surgery and in the presence of an anesthetic agent serve as a potent stimulus for arrhythmias. This sensitizing effect is limited mainly to gaseous anesthetics such as cyclopropane, halothane and methoxyflurane.

3. During surgery, manipulation and traction on the heart may produce arrhythmias. This is usually of little consequence as in most instances since the patient is rapidly placed on cardiopulmonary bypass. However, other surgical maneuvers may lead to rhythm disturbances that persist into the postoperative period. The atriotomy that must be performed for cannulation of the *vena cavae* may lead to atrial arrhythmias.Certain operations, such as the mustard procedure and closure of an atrial septal defect may damage the sinus node and atrial conduction pathways leading to a junctional rhythm postoperatively. Right or left bundle branch block or complete AV block may follow repair of a ventricular septal defect or aortic valve replacement.

ment of a suture, in which case the defect is largely irreversible, or from edema or hematoma compressing the conduction system, this frequently being reversible with the conduction abnormality improving days to weeks later.

4. Hypothermia may be used to reduce hypoxic tissue damage during open-heart surgery. While hypothermic, the patient typically develops sinus bradycardia which may progress to an escape junctional rhythm or ultimately asystole. However, on rewarming postoperatively, ventricular fibrillation may occur.

5. Metabolic abnormalities (Table 6.3) are frequently present in the postoperative period and may contribute to the devleopment of arrhythmias. Hypoxemia may occur as a result of hypoventilation, atelectasis or pulmonary edema. The reduced arterial oxygen tension may worsen myocardial ischemia leading to ventricular arrhythmias. Inadequate ventilation also produces an increase in arterial carbon dioxide tension and a fall in pH, both of which enhance automaticity. Poor tissue perfusion with excess lactic acid production may lead to metabolic acidosis. Hypokalemia is common following cardiac surgery and may be worsened by the administration of intravenous diuretics. This and other electrolyte disturbances, such as hypercalcemia, predispose to ventricular arrhythmias, especially when digitalis preparations have been administered.

6. Pericarditis may appear one to two weeks after surgery (post-pericardiotomy syndrome) and produce atrial fibrillation and other atrial arrhythmias. In the more immediate postoperative period, cardiac tamponade may result from bleeding into the pericardium and mediastinum. Initially, there is sinus tachycardia in response to a falling stroke volume and cardiac output, but ultimately ventricular fibrillation or asystole occurs if the problem is not recognized and corrected.

7. Digitalis preparations and diuretics are probably the most commonly prescribed drugs for patients with cardiac disease. Digitalis excess, especially in combination with hypokalemia induced by diuretic therapy is an important cause of arrhythmias in these patients following heart surgery.

TABLE 6.3

Metabolic Abnormalities Predisposing to Cardiac Arrhythmias

1. Hypoxia

2. Hypercapnia

3. Acid–base abnormalities

4. Electrolyte abnormalities

5. Hyperthyroidism

RECOGNITION AND TREATMENT OF SPECIFIC ARRHYTHMIAS

The cardiac arrhythmias which are frequently encountered in the postoperative period are summarized in Table 6.4. Their clinical significance and treatment are briefly discussed in the following paragraphs. The reader should refer to the appropriate chapters of the textbooks listed in the references for electrocardiographic examples of each arrhythmia.

ETOPIC BEATS

Premature atrial contractions occur frequently in the postoperative period, especially among patients with atrial enlargement. They may be an early sign of left ventricular failure which produces acute left atrial distention as the left ventricular filling pressure rises. Other predisposing factors include pericardial inflammation, hypoxia, and electrolyte abnormalities.

Premature atrial contractions rarely produce symptoms and usually can be treated conservatively with observation and a search for a correctable underlying cause. However, when they appear with increasing frequency, they may be the forerunner of atrial flutter or fibrillation. In such instances, digoxin along with quinidine or procainamide may be administered to prevent progression toward these tachyarrhythmias.

Premature ventricular contractions are the most commonly encountered arrhythmia in the postoperative period. Among patients who have undergone coronary artery bypass graft surgery, they may arise from persistent ischemia in areas of myocardium which were incompletely revascularized.

133

TABLE 6.4

Common Postoperative Arrhythmias

I. Ectopic Beats

    A. Premature atrial contractions
    B. Premature Junctional contractions
    C. Premature ventricular contractions

II. Tachyarrhythmias

    A. Sinus tachycardia
    B. Paroxysmal atrial tachycardia
    C. Atrial flutter
    D. Atrial fibrillation
    E. Junctional tachycardia
    F. Ventricular tachycardia
    G. Ventricular fibrillation

Hypoxemia, hypokalemia, the administration of sympathomimetic amines (bronchodilators, inotropic agents), and digitalis toxicity are other important etiologic factors.

Management should initially focus on identifying and correcting any of these predisposing problems. However, when premature ventricular contractions occur more frequently than five per minute, in pairs, or during the recovery phase of the preceding beat (R or T phenomenon), treatment with intravenous lidocaine is necessary.

TACHYARRHYTHMIAS

Sinus tachycardia is seen routinely following cardiac surgery and is a normal physiologic response the the pain and stress of the postoperative period. However, it may also reflect serious underlying problems, such as hypovolemia, sepsis, congestive heart failure, or cardiac tamponade. Although sinus tachycardia does not require special treatment, a thorough search should be made for these potentially underlying conditions.

Supraventricular tachycardia occurs most frequently among patients with congenital and valvular heart disease following cardiac surgery. This arrhythmia is easily tolerated by patients with otherwise healthy hearts. However, in patients with mitral stenosis or a prosthetic mitral valve, there may be a considerable fall in cardiac output at the higher heart rates. It may also worsen myocardial ischemia in patients with coronary artery disease.

Management should initially include the performance of several simple physiologic maneuvers (Table 6.5). Carotid sinus massage produces a relfex increase in vagal tone that may slow impulse conduction within the heart and terminate the arrhythmia. The Valsalva maneuver may also be effective by producing a similar in crease in vagal tone but is often impractical in the immediate postoperative period.

When these maneuvers fail, then pharmacologic agents must be used. Edrophonium is a short-acting inhibitor of cholinesterase. When this drug is given intravenously, acetylcholine accumulates at the postsynaptic parasympathetic nerve endings, elowing impulse conduction and often terminating the arrhythmia.

Raising the blood pressure is another effective way of treating supraventricular tachycardia, especially if the patient is hypotensive. Again, the

TABLE 6.5

TREATMENT OF SUPRAVENTRICULAR TACHYCARDIA

1. Carotid sinus massage
2. Valsalva maneuver
3. Edrophonium
4. Vasopressors
5. Propanolol
6. Digoxin or-
7. Electrical cardioversion

mechanism of action involves stimulation of the carotid sinus through the rise in blood pressure which in turn produces an increase in vagal tone. In practice, this is usually accomplished with intravenous administration of either phenylephrine or metaraminol.

When these measures fail, more specific antiarrhythmic drugs must be used. In otherwise healthy patients without evidence of congestive heart failure intravenous propranolol is frequently effective. However, following cardiac surgery, propranolol carries the potential danger of weakening myocardial contractility and reducing cardiac output. In this setting, intravenous digoxin is the drug of choice.

Paroxysmal atrial tachycardia is occasionally associated with atrioventricular block. This phenomenon most commonly occurs as a result of digitalis toxicity. Treatment should include withholding further digitalis preparations and correcting any potassium depletion that may be present.

Atrial flutter may occur postoperatively in patients with enlarged atria from either rheumatic or congenital heart disease. Characteristically, it is very responsive to electrical cardioversion, usually at low energy levels (25 to 50 watt-seconds). When there is any evidence of associated hemodynamic deterioration, this is the treatment of choice. However, atrial flutter is frequently a recurrent problem and drug therapy may ultimately be more effective. Initially, digoxin should be given intravenously to slow the ventricular response rate. Once this has been accomplished, quinidine may be given to convert or prevent further recurrences of the atrial flutter.

Atrial fibrillation is seen commonly in the postoperative period among all forms of heart disease. Predisposing factors include atrial enlargement, ischemia, surgical trauma to the atria, and pericardial inflammation.

Providing there is no hemodynamic compromise, treatment should initially focus on slowing the ventricular response with the administration of digoxin. Once the ventricular rate is controlled, quinidine may be given to convert the patient to sinus rhythm. In the presence of a very rapid ventricular rate and hemodynamic deterioration, electrical cardioversion may be required. Unfortunately, unlike atrial flutter, atrial fibrillation may require high energy levels or be altogether refractory, especially if it is long-standing or associated with massive atrial enlargement.

Ventricular tachycardia is most frequently encountered following cardiac surgery in patients with coronary artery disease. Typically, they have undergone coronary artery bypass graft surgery but have been left with areas of persistent myocardial ischemia. The problem may be compounded by co-existing hypoxemia or hypokalemia.

When the duration of ventricular tachycardia is brief and the blood pressure stable, intravenous lidocaine is the treatment of choice. This should be given as an initial bolus of 75 to 100 mg, followed by an infusion of from two to four mg per minute depending upon the patient's size and hemo-dynamic status. A second bolus of 75 mg may be necessary 30 minutes later to maintain the blood level continuously in the therapeutic range. If lidocaine proves ineffective in preventing recurrent episodes of ventricular tachycardia, then procainamide may be used. When ventricular tachycardia persists or produces significant hypotension, then electrical cardioversion becomes neces-sary and is usually effective at low levels (25 to 50 watt-seconds).

Ventricular fibrillation is characterized by rapid irregular depolariza-tion of the ventricles with loss of effective ventricular contraction. Underlying etiologies are essentially the same as for ventricular tachycardia. If the patient is to be saved, treatment must be instituted immediately in the form of cardio-pulmonary resuscitation and electrical defibrillation.

REFERENCES

1.   Angelini P, Feldman MI, Lupschanowski R, et al. Cardiac arrhythmias during and after heart surgery: diagnosis and management. Prog Cardio-vas Dis 16: 469-95, 1974.

2.   Smith R, Grossman W, Johnson L, et al. Arrhythmias following valve replacement. Circulation 45: 1018-23, 1972.

3.   Gomez G, Gonzalez F, Adams C, et al. Electrocardiographic findings after open heart surgery in children. Amer Heart J 64: 730-8, 1962.

4.   DeSanctis R, Block P, Hutter AM. Tachyarrhythmias in myocardial infarction. Circulation 45: 681-702, 1972.

5.   Marriott HJL, Sander IA. Criteria, old and new, for differentiating between ectopic ventricular beats and aberrant ventricular conduction in the presence of atrial fibrillation. Prog Cardiovas Dis 9: 18, 1966.

6.   Marriott HJL, Myerburg RJ. Recognition and treatment of cardiac arrhythmias and conduction distrubances. In: JW, Hurst and RG, Logue Eds, The Heart, 3rd ed, New York, McGraw-Hill, 1974, p 502-58.

7.   Schamroth L. The Disorders of Heart Rhythm. London, Blackwell Scientific, 1971.

8.   Friedberg CK. Diseases of the Heart, 3rd ed, Philadelphia, WB Saunders Co, 1966.

INDEX

Resistance, definition, 48
Respiratory failure, 123
Rest pain, 56
Risk factors, in post-MI patient, 91

Sarcolemma, 114
Sarcomere, 114
Sarcoplasmic reticulum, 114
Secretions, pulmonary, 124
Sector scanner two-dimensional ultrasound, 17
Shock lung. *See* Adult respiratory syndrome
Sinus tachycardia, 134
Smoking, and pulmonary complications, 123
Sonar, 3
Sound beam, width of, 5
Sound waves, 4
ST segment depression, 43
Steady state, 26
Stress, circulatory response to, test of, 58–59
Stress testing. *See* Exercise electrocardiography
Strip-chart recorder, in echocardiography, 5
Stroke
    causes, 69
    completed, 63
    noninvasive screening for, 63–77
    risk factors, 65
    types, 63
Stroke volume, exercise and, 81, 83
Supraventricular tachycardia, 135–136
Systemic hypothermia, in myocardial preservation, 113
Systole, 7

T-system, 114
Tachyarrhythmias, 134–137
Tachycardia. *See* Tachyarrhythmias
Target MET level, 102
Team approach, in patient education, 90
Thallium 201, in exercise perfusion scintigraphy, 39
Therapy, exercise electrocardiographic evaluation of, 22
Thoracic outlet compression, 58
Time-motion mode. *See* M-mode echocardiogram
Tissue necrosis, 56
Transducer, placement of, in linear array two-dimensional ultrasound, 15
    in m-mode echocardiography, 4
Transient ischemic attacks, 63
Trauma, and acute arterial vascular disease, 57

Treadmill test. *See* Exercise electrocardiography
Two-dimensional ultrasound, 11–17
   linear array system, 13-15, 16
      applications, 14, 16
      limitations, 13
   mechanical sector scanner, 17
   phased array system, 15

Ultrasonic nebulizers, in postsurgical pulmonary therapy, 126
Ultrasonography, 1
Ultrasound
   in cardiovascular diagnosis, 3–17
   Doppler. *See* Doppler ultrasound
   one-dimensional. *See* M-mode echocardiogram
   two-dimensional, 11–17
      linear array system, 13–15, 16
      mechanical sector scanner, 17
      phased array system, 15
United States Air Force protocol, for symptom-limited stress test, 101–102

Valsalva maneuver, in supraventricular tachycardia, 135
Vasopressors, in supraventricular tachycardia, 135–136
Veins, Doppler signal components, 51
Velocity, definition, 48
Velocity signal analysis, 54
Venous occlusion plethysmography, 55
Ventricular fibrillation, 137
   in myocardial preservation, 113
Ventricular pressure curves, during mitral valve motion, 9
Ventricular tachycardia, 136–137
$\dot{V}O_2$. *See* Oxygen consumption

Warm-up exercises, 106
Work capacity, electrocardiographic assessment of, 22

Xenon washout, 58